America on Foot

ALSO BY KERRY SEGRAVE
AND FROM MCFARLAND

*Suntanning in 20th Century America* (2005)

*Endorsements in Advertising: A Social History* (2005)

*Women and Smoking in America, 1880 to 1950* (2005)

*Foreign Films in America: A History* (2004)

*Lie Detectors: A Social History* (2004)

*Product Placement in Hollywood Films: A History* (2004)

*Piracy in the Motion Picture Industry* (2003)

*Jukeboxes: An American Social History* (2002)

*Vending Machines: An American Social History* (2002)

*Age Discrimination by Employers* (2001)

*Shoplifting: A Social History* (2001)

*Movies at Home: How Hollywood Came to Television* (1999)

*American Television Abroad: Hollywood's Attempt to
Dominate World Television* (1998)

*Tipping: An American Social History of Gratuities* (1998)

*American Films Abroad: Hollywood's Domination of
the World's Movie Screens from the 1890s to the Present* (1997)

*Baldness: A Social History* (1996)

*Policewomen: A History* (1995)

*Payola in the Music Industry: A History, 1880–1991* (1994)

*The Sexual Harassment of Women
in the Workplace, 1600 to 1993* (1994)

*Drive-in Theaters: A History from Their Inception in 1933* (1992)

*Women Serial and Mass Murderers: A Worldwide Reference,
1580 through 1990* (1992)


BY KERRY SEGRAVE AND LINDA MARTIN
AND FROM MCFARLAND

*The Continental Actress: European Film Stars of the Postwar Era;
Biographies, Criticism, Filmographies, Bibliographies* (1990)

*The Post Feminist Hollywood Actress: Biographies and
Filmographies of Stars Born After 1939* (1990)

# America on Foot

*Walking and Pedestrianism in the 20th Century*

KERRY SEGRAVE

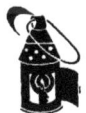

McFarland & Company, Inc., Publishers
*Jefferson, North Carolina, and London*

LIBRARY OF CONGRESS CATALOGUING-IN-PUBLICATION DATA

Segrave, Kerry, 1944–
    America on foot : walking and pedestrianism in the 20th century / Kerry Segrave.
        p.    cm.
    Includes bibliographical references and index.

    ISBN 0-7864-2559-8 (softcover : 50# alkaline paper) ∞

    1. Walking—United States—History.   2. Pedestrians—Legal status, laws, etc.—United States.   I. Title.
    GV1071.S44    2006
    796.510973—dc22                                            2006004470

British Library cataloguing data are available

©2006 Kerry Segrave. All rights reserved

*No part of this book may be reproduced or transmitted in any form or by any means, electronic or mechanical, including photocopying or recording, or by any information storage and retrieval system, without permission in writing from the publisher.*

Cover photograph ©2006 Image State

Manufactured in the United States of America

*McFarland & Company, Inc., Publishers
   Box 611, Jefferson, North Carolina 28640
      www.mcfarlandpub.com*

# Contents

*Preface* 1

1. The Years to 1900 3
2. Famous Walkers 13
3. Nobody Walks 25
4. Long Distance Walking 30
5. The Nature of Walking 39
6. Instructing the Masses in How to Walk 48
7. Clubs, Governments, and Images 66
8. Benefits of Walking — Mental and Psychological 78
9. Benefits of Walking — Health and Medical 86
10. Walking Reborn as a Trendy Exercise 98
11. Marketers Target Walking 110
12. Psychological Aspects of Walking 122
13. Walking by the Numbers 130
14. Pedestrians Versus Cars 136
15. Regulating Pedestrians, to 1950 151
16. Regulating Pedestrians, 1950–2005 168
17. Conclusion 181

*Notes* 185
*Bibliography* 199
*Index* 209

# Preface

Walking was not an activity people undertook out of choice until around the 1700s. Prior to that, walking had been a necessity for all but the wealthier class. When the literary segment of European society took strongly to the long, excursive walk in the 1800s, it was a trend that transferred only partly to America. In the United States, distance walking was more likely to be a series of races, complete with prizes and spectators, and held on indoor tracks. But some of the promenading found in Europe did come to the U.S., especially in the larger cities, as did some aspects of the leisurely, contemplative walk, an activity to bring one closer to Nature, to stimulate thought processes, and to lead to intellectual discoveries and creations.

Thus, in the America of 1900 walking was not concerned with speed of the stroll, outside of races, or heart beat rate, or of health benefits, nor was it even thought of as an exercise. As the 1900s passed, walkers declined in numbers, as did attention paid to the subject, until there was a revival of interest in walking from the late 1970s onward, a revival due to people coming late to a fitness boom that had started in the 1960s and for whom fitness activities such as running were too strenuous.

But with the revival of walking came a reinvention of the activity. All of its former intellectual, contemplative, and observational qualities were simply banished, no longer mentioned, as walking was redefined as having only instrumental value. Numbers and mathematic equations relating, for example, to target heart rate and calorie burn rate became preoccupations. Nature was removed when indoor walking at malls became popular. Special shoes were sold to participants, as were pedometers and books and articles which purported to teach them how to walk. Substituted for the mental benefits of walking that earlier proponents of the activity touted were an increasingly growing set of health benefits, which at times bordered on the miraculous. At the same time, as walking became popular in the late 1900s, the standard of what was necessary in order to be classed as a regular walker or a fitness walker underwent a steady lowering of the bar.

The second part of the book deals with the pedestrian — the walker who interacted with vehicles. Automobiles have largely been responsible for the decline of walking in America, and the 1900s was a century in which the walker lost out almost always to the car as the automobile came to dominate all land use and land planning decisions. The century was one in which a continuous effort was made to regulate and control pedestrians in order that vehicles could move more smoothly and quickly. Despite the overwhelming advantages the vehicle possessed in confrontations with pedestrians — from its size, speed and lethality, to traffic signal timing cycles, to right turns on red lights, to lenient treatment of offending motorists — the walker was more likely the one to be blamed in the event of an accident. This, then, is the story of walking and pedestrianism in 20th-century America.

# 1
# The Years to 1900

> "A pedestrian seems in this country [England] to be a sort of beast of passage — stared at, pitied, suspected and shunned by everybody who meets him."
> Carl Philip Moritz, 1782
>
> "With women, half of the ill health and all defects in gait and figure arise from our false methods of locomotion."
> Anonymous, 1890s

Walking was always such a natural method of getting around, and often the only way, that it was not given much thought or attention in the early years. It was not until the 1800s that walking first took on any faddish aspects — as in the long walks and hikes so favored by the literary set and others of that era; that is, people went for long walks when they did not have to do so and they did so because it was felt that walking bestowed certain benefits on them. But it was the 1900s before the faddish aspects became prevalent, when articles and books were written on the topic of how to walk and special clothing was designed for the activity. It was also in the 1900s that pedestrianism was truly born — the person in the crowded urban centers moving a relatively short distance, say, from a parking lot to an office or shopping area downtown. Walking became an inherently more dangerous activity at the same time as the age of pedestrianism was marked by the arrival of the car culture; the automobile proved itself to be the natural enemy of the person on foot.

According to an estimate of anthropologist Robert Briffault, early man — a hunter — walked an average of 20 miles a day. In contrast, when a Gallup poll surveyed the physical habits of Canadians in September 1955, it concluded that during that autumn month the average citizen walked a fraction less than two miles a day.[1] Benefits from walking, both physical and mental, were attributed to the activity as far back as ancient times. Dr. Arthur Patch McKinlay, emeritus professor of Latin at UCLA remarked that walking was described by the Greek writer Pliny the Elder (A.D. 23–79) as one of the "Medicines of the Will," meaning you had to have willpower enough to take them. One prominent Greek physician who mentioned walking was Hippocrates (circa 469–399 B.C.). In one chapter of his book, he mentioned walking 40 times in connection with digestive diseases. He prescribed brisk walks, short walks, early morning walks, after-dinner walks, and night walks. Early morning walks were recommended for emotional disturbances; morning and evening walks for overly sensitive people; brisk strolls to reduce hallucinations, to reduce weight, and to maintain a trim figure.[2]

In classical Athens, walking was part of the discipline of two philosophical schools—the peripatetic and the stoic. The origin of "peripatetic" was the Greek word *peripatos*, which meant "to walk about." Aristotle (384–322 B.C.), who founded the Peripatetic School, instructed his students as he strolled with them through the shaded grove of the Lyceum. Philosophers at that famous school had all of their discourses while walking. Stoics took their name from the word *stoa*, meaning "roofed colonnade." Stoas were built to screen shops and pedestrians from the sun and it was in the shade of a stoa that Zeno of Citium and other Stoic philosophers of the third century B.C. held forth.[3]

Researchers Simon Breines and William Dean observed that in ancient Athens the busiest place in the city was the agora, the "gathering place," which was an open public space located below the Acropolis. It was a pedestrian area in downtown Athens with markets, shrines and government buildings. Today, many Spanish cities have a public space for walking called a *rambla*—from the Arabic word *ramla*, meaning "dry riverbed." In the evening, it was the custom for the populace to stroll along the rambla, or avenue, chatting with friends. Also, the rambla provided parents with the opportunity to place their eligible daughters on view. World famous were the Ramblus in Barcelona, Spain, and a wooded area called the Ramble in New York City's Central Park.[4]

From the time of the earliest cities until the 19th century, argued Breines and Dean, urban planners took care to scale the city to humans and to their natural ability for movement on their own two feet. By the late 1900s London was about 650 times as large as the area covered by medieval London. Rome, when enclosed by the Aurelian Wall in A.D. 274, was little more than five square miles. Still, the city was felt to be congested. Due to that congestion in Rome's streets, Julius Caesar, in one of his first acts upon coming to power in 49 B.C., moved to ban carts and chariots from the city between sunrise and sunset. In Pompeii, the city's forum was a pedestrian mall, closed to wheeled traffic by the use of bollards. The medieval street, usually winding and narrow, served principally as a pedestrian route. Since the needs of wheeled traffic were secondary it made sense to let streets follow nature's contours rather than to artificially straighten them. "With footpower as the principal means of movement, walking distance served as an effective limit on urban expansion," said Breines and Dean; and "Medieval street patterns tended to be circular and radial. The straight avenues of the gridiron system came later as a response to the demands of fast-traveling, horse-drawn carriages." In the view of these researchers the automobile stole the street, with the street reduced to the single basic function of a passageway and storage area for motor vehicles. The pedestrian of the past, they believed, was better off than the pedestrian of today, Caesar's ban on cart and chariot traffic in the daytime in Rome showing a concern for pedestrians not usually found in the modern world. "Few public officials now even think about pedestrians," concluded Breines and Dean. "The social life and activity found in the streets of classical Athens, fourth-century Antioch and the medieval city are rarely found in modern cities; we are the poorer for this." The Roman soldier of ancient times was said to have walked an average of 21 miles a day, with full pack.[5]

Speculation was that too much walking may have led to the English defeat at the hands of William the Conqueror back in 1066 at the Battle of Hastings. The Saxons of King Harold covered 200 miles on foot to London where they paused briefly before going on to Hastings. They covered that 200 miles in an unknown period of time; modern estimates placed it at four to 10 days. In 1956, to find out how much that march might have affected the Saxons, six members of the Surrey Walking Club in England got into chain mail, picked up the full packs and weapons the ancient soldiers might have toted, and set off. They took six hours and 14 minutes to cover 20 miles the first day. By the end of that day they'd had enough and canceled the remainder of the planned march.[6]

Noted historian Lewis Mumford observed that streets were originally made wide and straight so the military could march on them more easily; and wide streets offered better protection against assault from within, compared to narrow and/or winding streets. "In the medieval town the upper classes and the lower classes had jostled together on the street, in the marketplace, as they did in the cathedral: the rich might ride on horseback, but they must wait for the poor man with his bundle or the blind beggar groping with his stick to get out of the way," wrote Mumford. However, with the development of the wide avenue, the dissociation of the upper and the lower classes took place in the city itself: "The rich drive;

the poor walk. The rich roll along the axis of the grand avenue; the poor are off-center, in the gutter; and eventually a special strip is provided for the ordinary pedestrian, the sidewalk." According to Mumford the needs of wheeled traffic became urgent in the 17th century. An 18th-century writer by the name of Mercier said, "The threatening wheels of the overbearing rich drive as rapidly as ever over stones stained with the blood of their unhappy victims." Mumford added that such a sentiment did not exaggerate the danger because in France, the stagecoach, introduced in the 17th century, killed more people annually than did the railroad that followed it.[7]

In New York in 1676 (New Amsterdam at that time), when the town was over a century old, only a few streets had been paved with cobblestones and provided with a gutter in the center, but not with sidewalks. Researcher Bernard Rudofsky noted it was no wonder that people did not feel like walking in the streets after nightfall. There were no streetlights; therefore the city board ordered that "all and every of the housekeepers within the city shall put lights in their windows fronting the streets." When that method of illumination proved to be of little value, the board then decreed that every seventh house was to set out on the street a candle-lit lantern on a pole, with the expenses to be shared by the people in the six adjoining houses. Sometime in the 1690s New York prohibited the dumping of refuse in the street—presumably removing one impediment to walking after dark—and the city decreed that no swine be allowed "to go or range in any of the streets." The New York Corporation voted as its first budget for street cleaning in 1696 a grand total of $20.[8]

In her book on walking and English culture, Anne Wallace explained that the transportation revolution, beginning in the mid 18th century, affected walking in several ways by the early 19th century. First, it altered the socioeconomic content of walking by making fast, cheap travel available to the laboring classes, increasing the attractiveness of travel in general and removing the long-standing implications that walking was undertaken out of necessity and/or poverty and denoted vagrancy. Walking must have once been the only mode of travel available to the mass of humanity. Until roughly the middle of the 18th century there were only two alternatives: the riding horse and the animal-drawn wheeled vehicle. Roads were extremely poor quality until then with coach travel being very slow (three to nine miles per hour) and very rough.[9]

Wallace pointed out that in the time of Jonathan Swift (1667–1745), the vast majority of his contemporaries were villagers who rarely in their lifetime traveled further than a day's walking distance from home. During the Middle Ages in England, Wallace wrote, "The greatest suspicion of all fell on pedestrians, whose mode of travel proclaimed their poverty and therefore the greater probability of their being wanderers with some illicit or economically disruptive motive." Walking was the cheapest kind of travel, but also the slowest, most physically demanding, and most dangerous. Those walking on the road were likely to be among the economically discontented and disenfranchised who had little or no choice as to their mode of travel — beggars, fleeing serfs, dishonest pedlars, or thieves. Right through the 1700s, declared Wallace, "It was supposed that no man of substance would ever walk, except with a gun over his shoulder, and that everyone who tramped the roads was either a footpad [thief *without* a horse; a highwayman was a thief *with* a horse] or a pauper.... It was not till the early nineteenth century when the highways were improved and robbers were less numerous, that walking became the pleasure and pastime of all classes." Special difficulties existed for female walkers because of the implications of sexual promiscuity. Partly that came from rural lower-class courtship patterns. "Walking out" with someone in that time period had the same meaning as going steady or being engaged had in the modern era. Also, walking out was often understood to include sexual intercourse. Implications from that earlier time can still be found in the current term "streetwalker" (the lowest class of prostitute).[10]

Carl Philip Moritz, a German clergyman traveling as a walker in England in 1782, said, "A pedestrian seems in this country to be a sort of beast of passage — stared at, pitied, suspected and shunned by everybody who meets him." Before the transportation revolution, concluded Wallace, "walking as travel meant poverty, alienation from society whether for legal or extra-legal reasons, possible moral turpitude, and probably danger to the individuals and communities touched by the act." Richard Pyke, describing the Italian leg of the Grand Tour (late in the 18th century) asserted, "One thing the traveler never did — walk. Only outlaws and madmen walked; it was considered neither safe nor a pleasure." Such travel advice changed around the turn of the 19th century when William Wordsworth took his pedestrian tour, and by 1818, travel guides, said Wallace, commended the "pedestrian tour," whereas in 1788, travel guides did not envision foot travel, except where no other kind was possible. As travel became cheap for the masses in the early part of the 19th century, walking became a matter of choice. It became a positive choice and since the common person did not need to travel by foot it followed that walking travelers did not necessarily have to be poor. England's parliament pushed for cheap rail fares that allowed laborers to live outside of city centers — that is, to live more than walking distance away from their employment. The railway, said Wallace, "became for urban labourers the everyday passage between work and home that the footpath was for rural labourers."[11]

Throughout the 19th century, added Wallace, there was an increase in the amount of deliberate excursive walking, especially by the relatively well-to-do and educated classes, with conspicuous examples set by Wordsworth and Samuel Taylor Coleridge. Thomas De Quincey developed a routine of walking 70 to 100 miles per week, while John Keats walked 642 miles during his 1818 tour of the Lakes and Scotland, with the idea that such tramping would "give me more experience, rub off more Prejudice ... identifying finer scenes, load me with grander Mountains." A general wave of pedestrian touring began in the late 18th century, of which the literary men mentioned above were part. By the middle of the 19th century deliberate excursive walking had become identified with the intellectual classes, but was not limited to them. Some of them reportedly walked 25 or 30 miles a day for most of their lives. However, those people regarded their long walks as quite different from the fad for long walks that started in the U.S. around 1850. Excursive walking was done at a relatively leisurely pace with a view to getting in touch with nature, inspiring the creative process in the many literary people in that movement, and so forth. On the other hand, in America the fad was all about running up large numbers—distance covered—competitions, and winning bets and/or prizes. It was what emerged when the activity of walking long distances was reworked to suit and to reflect the buccaneer capitalism of the day.[12]

Historian Penelope Corfield looked at walking the city streets in late 18th century England and concluded the experience was mostly a pleasant one. She argued that custom and convention in England endorsed the accessibility of the streets to all age and social groups and to both sexes. And walking, therefore, was not just a utilitarian necessity but a pleasant form of informal entertainment in its own right, with the urban promenade being the occasion for people to view the sights and each other, to see and be seen. Corfield called it an integral part of social life. In many cities, the main occasions for social walking were on Sundays, on holidays, and during special festivities. Meanwhile, in London and in certain spas and resorts elsewhere, fashionable society promenaded daily in the season, both in the mornings and the afternoons, weather permitting. Reported a visitor to Bath, England, in May 1767, "I was an hour and three quarters on my legs. Oh, my poor legs! They reproach me for it to this very minute."[13]

Corfield argued that in that period there was a marked development and formalization of special areas for the purpose of communal walking, especially in spas, resorts, and leisure cities, but copied in many other urban centers. New streets were laid out and designated as "parades," "walks," and "promenades." Town squares also represented the victory of formalized public space over development density. Parks were popular places for the activity, with the social promenade enjoyed by all classes of society. In this period, concluded Corfield, a growing number of coaches and carriages began to usurp space and take priority: "Pedestrian areas were therefore increasingly separated from driving zones, being demarcated by posts or by raised sections of paving."[14]

An editorial in the *Times* of London in September 1930 referred to an article exactly 100 years earlier in the same newspaper about how dangerous it was to be a pedestrian in London in 1830, what with all the wheeled traffic and carriage drivers who complained about pedestrians not looking where they were going. In 1830 it was said that if a considerable extension of sidewalks took place in most of the main streets the trouble would be over and pedestrians would be safe. Said the 1930 editor, "The streets of London have always been very dangerous to pedestrians. In Tudor times the chief danger lay in rogues, vagabonds, discharged servants, starving agricultural workers, etc. In the 18th century, the greatest danger was dirt. By 1830, traffic had taken first place, to hold it ever since."[15]

Prodigious walking feats were often reported in earlier times. Covering long distances on foot was common in the frontier days of North America. In October 1808, trapper John Coulter, after an encounter with Indians left him without equipment, walked 200 miles to the nearest fort. It took him eight days. Robert Campbell, of the Hudson's Bay Company, covered around 3,000 miles in a little over six months in 1852–1853.[16]

When researcher Davis Scobey investigated walking in 19th century New York, he concluded that bourgeois New Yorkers of the Victorian era loved to promenade throughout most of that century. They made seeing and being seen — in public and in motion — an integral part of sociability and a badge of inclusion within the metropolitan gentry. The first phase, he declared, came in the late 1820s and early 1830s, the era of the Erie Canal and the creation of a fashionable residential and shopping district around the uptown reaches of Broadway. "It was then that promenading became a defining ritual for the city's bourgeois elite," said Scobey. In the 1820s, Broadway became the city's main thoroughfare and most fashionable promenade, where the elites flocked to shop and show themselves. A second phase took place in the late 1850s and 1860s, when Wall Street won control of national finance and then with a guidebook, reporting in the mid–1880s, "Fifth avenue is the fashionable promenade." Scobey argued there was dramatically less evidence of formal promenading beginning in the 1890s.[17]

However, the real focus on walking in America in the latter half of the 19th century and into the early part of the 20th century was in long-distance walking of all sorts. Before the Civil War, young lower-class men earned money by challenging people to walking contests of all types. When the Civil War brought together soldiers from all classes, competitive walking was gentrified and a nationwide movement known as "pedestrianism," involving organized competitive walking, took hold. Fans of the events formed clubs and sponsored contests, wrote journalist Kerry Pechter. During the movement's heyday, the old Madison Square Garden in New York was the site of six-day footraces that drew thousands of spectators and paid winners up to $50,000. The best known pedestrian from the era was Edward Payson Weston, who once walked, on a wager, to Abraham Lincoln's inauguration. In 1867 he walked 1,326 miles from Portland, Maine, to Chicago in 26 days. Once, he walked exactly 100 miles in 22 hours, 19 minutes and 10 seconds. In 1909, at the age of 70, Weston walked from New York to San Francisco, covering the 3,895 miles in 104 days and seven hours. When he was 88, in 1927, he was struck and crippled (while out walking) by a New York City taxicab. Pechter declared pedestrianism lost favor in the 1890s amid charges of fixed races, and amateur cross-country walking faded out by about 1915.[18]

If prizes were sometimes large and crowds sometimes huge at walking matches the average event was far more modest. An audience that numbered around 200, mostly women, was present on December 24, 1888 at Hazard's Pavilion in Los Angeles for the commencement of a six-day walking match. A track eight feet wide with a covering of sawdust six inches deep was arranged around the hall; 14 laps equaled a mile. Nine contestants started the contest, all men, and none were said to appear to be over 28 years of age. The race was kicked off by a short address from Mayor Bryson, who said, in part, "Endurance, strength and courage are elements essential to success in all the callings of life, particularly in a pedestrian contest." Bryson said he had been told it was the first incidence of a six-day contest in the history of Los Angeles. After the contest's first hour, the three leaders had covered, respectively, eight, seven, and seven miles.[19] When a week-long walking match ended in Detroit in April 1894, it was declared a financial flop, although two of the walkers covered the required 425 miles. After figuring up the income and expenses, it was found that the walkers' share was just $14.32.[20] For some of his marathon walking tours Weston had a schedule wherein he would walk 36 miles a day from Tuesday to Saturday, rest on Sundays, and walk 50 miles on Mondays. So popular was Weston during his heyday that he got press coverage around the United States almost every day as journalists reported on his daily doings.[21]

In the years prior to 1900, walking was just something people went out and did. There were next to no articles that proposed to tell people how to do it; there were very few mentions of health benefits from the activity. But there were somewhat more numerous mentions about the mental benefits. One exception was an 1883 piece directed at women, which declared a new fashion in female walking had been invented at the West End Hotel in New York. A journalist described it as "too lovely for anything" and described it as of a series of carefully balanced steps, "first on one foot and then on the other, and has the charming effect of bringing every part of the body into what may be called the very poetry of motion." Continuing along the same line, the account enthused, "The arms swing gracefully from side to side, forming one unbroken, waving line of beauty. The neck bends into the most perfect arches; the chest is expanded in the most natural manner, and the shoulders are set off at the utmost perfection." All *that* was accomplished, it was asserted, by the women "persistently wearing the tightest of tight shoes."[22]

Millicent Arrowpoint reported in 1895 about a new walking cure for physical defects then said to be popular in London, England. It was promulgated by an unnamed male professor who discovered that, "with women, half the ill health and all defects in gait and figure arise from our false methods of locomotion." To walk properly, he said, was to hold and move the body so that every muscle was exactly balanced and employed, and on that principle he guaranteed to bring any woman's figure "back into lines of strength and grace." Reportedly, he had a long list of aristocratic clients. Those wealthy women received a half-hour session at his home/office where, he said, "They are all threading the mazes of intricate patterns, stars, circles, angles and squares, marked out on the floor." Other of those students were simply set to walking up and down a long straight line, counting "one, two, three" at every step to the time marked by a big music box playing in one corner of the room. When a pupil's 30 minute session was over, the professor gave her a piece of folded paper on which was drawn a new diagram, which she was expected to practice at home for two hours every day. According to the professor, ill-fitting shoes, careless habits, and forcing children to walk too early "lends to women their unsightly gait, that is not at all improved by the awkward heavy skirts and the corsets they are obliged to don." Thus they had thrown their bodies out of alignment and harmony and to restore that equilibrium the professor taught those unfortunate women "these processes of self-locomotion."[23]

Another advice and health-benefit article declared that a "never-failing cure for nervous headache" was the simple act of walking backward. The relief provided was said to be "always certain and generally speedy," with 10 minutes being the maximum time before relief arrived. Besides curing nervous headache, the account claimed there was no better way to learn to walk well and gracefully forward than by practicing the activity backward and "a half hour of it once a day will do wonders toward improving the gait of any woman."[24]

As early as 1896 a reporter declared — prematurely — that long-distance walking was out of fashion and out of favor. In his view, the arrival of the bicycle craze was responsible for the decrease in walking even though "the cyclist misses a great deal, in addition to having chosen the less health-giving pastime. In the cultivation of sound lungs and broad shoulders the pedestrian has no rival." Foreshadowing sentiments that would be heard a century later, this journalist remarked there were peculiar deterrents to systematic walking in large towns, chief of which was "the ring of dull and sometimes dirty suburbs, which has to be penetrated before the open is reached and actual pleasure commences."[25]

Throughout history, many famous people have been well known as walkers and/or enthusiastic proponents of the activity.

# 2

# Famous Walkers

*"I like to go by myself. Nature is company enough for me. I cannot see the wit of walking and talking at the same time."*
                              William Hazlitt (1778–1830).

*"'Tis the best of humanity that goes out to walk."*
                              Ralph Waldo Emerson (1803–1882).

*"Only those thoughts that come by walking have any value."*
                              Friedrich Wilhelm Nietzsche (1844–1900).

*"You never heard of anyone doing away with himself after a long walk."*
                              George M. Cohan (1878–1942).

Hippocrates (circa 469–399 B.C.), the ancient Greek physician, asserted, "Walking is man's best medicine." Plato (428–347 B.C.) said, tongue in cheek, that a walk "would almost cure a guilty conscience," while the Jewish physician Maimonides, who practiced in a Cairo suburb during the 12th century, said, in referring to the laxative effect of walking, "A person should walk prior to the meal until his body begins to be warmed." Two centuries later, the Dutch humanist Erasmus agreed with Maimonides when he advised, "Before supper walk a little; after supper do the same." Leonardo da Vinci (1452–1519), a great walker himself, planned a city with elevated streets for pedestrians in order to isolate and protect them from cart traffic.[1] Francis Bacon (1561–1626) was said to have extolled walking for health, while William Shakespeare (1564–1616) was described as preferring to walk on footpaths rather than roadways and as being one of many who did a lot of their thinking while walking. Ben Johnson (1572–1637) was a great walker who once tramped from London to Scotland. Another prodigious walker was Thomas Hobbes (1588–1679).

Jonathan Swift (1667–1745) walked ten miles a day. One of the few dissenters was William Congreve (1670–1745), who said, "I nauseate walking; 'tis a country diversion." Of course that was before the idea that walking might be a pleasure, even a profitable pastime took strong hold in the early to mid 19th century. Early prodigious walkers (those who walked by choice and not from necessity), such as the ones mentioned above, engaged in the activity before the activity had many followers.[2]

Johann Sebastian Bach (1685–1750), while still a boy, once hiked 200 miles to hear the renowned Buxtehude play the organ. William Penn (1644–1718) made a famous "walking purchase" from the Delaware Indians after his commissioners concluded a 1686 treaty. Under that treaty it was agreed that the Delawares would relinquish all the land between the Delaware and Lehigh rivers from a southerly boundary at what became Bethlehem, Pennsylvania, "north to the farthest point that a man could walk in three days." Samuel Johnson (1709–1784) was also described as a great walker. Thomas Jefferson (1743–1826) remarked in 1776, "Of all exercises walking is the best." He was an enthusiastic walker all of his life. While composing the talks that gave rise to Methodism, religious teacher John Wesley (1703–1791) found that brisk walks of 20 and 30 miles a day put "spirit into his sermons."[3]

Jean-Jacques Rousseau (1712–1778) observed, "Never have I thought so much, never have I realized my own existence so much, been so much alive, been so much myself if I may say so, as in those journeys which I have made alone and on foot. Walking has something in it which animates and heightens my ideas: I can scarcely think when I stay in one place; my body must be set a-going if my mind is to work." To that he added, "The sight of the country, the succession of beautiful scenes, the great breeze, the good appetite, the health which I gain by walking, the getting away from inns, the escape from everything which reminds me of my lack of independence, from everything which reminds me of my unlucky fate...."[4]

Charles Lamb (1775–1834) was a city walker who also took delight in night walks around the city. Thomas De Quincey (1785–1859) said one of the things he looked forward to "was on Saturday nights, after I had taken opium, to wander forth, without much regarding the direction or the distance, to all the markets, and other parts of London, whither the poor resort on a Saturday night for laying out their wages.... Some of these rambles led me to great distances; for an opium eater is too happy to observe the motion of time."[5]

Edward Sackville West, De Quincey's biographer, said that De Quincey, aged 22, met Samuel Taylor Coleridge for the first time at a dinner party and was so excited by the events of the day that he decided to walk back to Bristol through the night. Of those night walks, De Quincey observed, "I seemed to myself in solitary possession of the whole sleeping country." What he liked about those solitary night rambles was "to trace the course of the evening through its household hieroglyphics from the windows which I passed or saw..." West declared those walks gave a lively satisfaction to the imagination of De Quincey, and that the walking habit remained with him until the end of his life. De Quincey believed the night walks promoted the dreaming faculty. His neighbors, recounted West, "seeing the tiny figure flit past their windows, with body, head, and arms held rigid and only the legs flickering in rapid movements, thought him mad, but he did not care." Night walks through the streets of London were especially important to De Quincey during the period when he was an opium addict, around 1813 to 1815. Later, said West, he looked to nocturnal walks to bring relief from a state of depression, but, "even these only served to renew impressions which, once so bright and keen with pleasurable sensations, now increased his sense of difference by a slow film of sadness."[6] In *Confessions of an English Opium Eater*, De Quincey declared it was possible to walk away from a variety of problems, "I have generally found that, if you are in quest of some certain escape from Philistines of whatever class—sheriff-officers, bores, no matter what—the surest refuge is to be found amongst hedgerows and fields."[7]

John Keats (1795–1821) was 22 when he accepted the invitation of his friend Charles Brown, who was 31 and also a writer, to undertake a walking tour of about 2,000 miles through northern England and Scotland, with a side trip to Northern Ireland. They were to leave in June 1818 and finish the trip three months later at the northern extremity of Scotland after starting out at Lancaster. Wrote Keats, "I purpose within a month to put my knapsack at my back and make a pedestrian tour through the North of England, and part of Scotland—to make a sort of Prologue to the Life I intend to pursue—that is to write, study and to see all of Europe at the lowest expense." In fact, he did not complete the trip. After starting on June 24 he caught a throat infection on the Isle of Mull and had to turn back on August 7, having reached Inverness. Just a few years later Keats died of consumption at the age of 25. Carol Kyros Walker, his biographer, stated, "The walking tour proved critical in the somatic profile of Keats. His condition was never quite the same afterward. His defenses were permanently down."[8]

Thomas Carlyle (1795–1881) was described as an "untiring walker" who often trekked alone in the quiet of the moors and the hills. His longest walk was one of 54 miles. All of the great naturalists were habitual walkers, including Gilbert White (1720–1793) and Izaak Walton (1593–1683) in England and John Muir (1838–1914) in the U.S. John James Audubon (1785–1851) could, and often did, walk 100 miles in two days.[9] William Wordsworth (1770–1850) was another prodigious walker. De Quincey commented that Wordsworth must have walked 175,000 or 180,000 miles in total, a mode of exertion, said De Quincey, "which to him stood in the stead of alcohol and all stimulants whatsoever to the animal spirits; to which, indeed, he was indebted for a life of unclouded happiness, and we for much of what is most excellent in his writings." Wordsworth was said to have walked 14 miles a day just to pick up his mail. He and Samuel Taylor Coleridge blocked out "The Rime of the Ancient Mariner" while they were on a walking tour in Somerset. When a traveler asked Wordsworth's servant to show him the writer's study she replied, "Here is his library, but his study is out of doors."[10]

Around 1785, as a teenager, Wordsworth began to write poetry and, according to his biographer, Hunter Davies, most of his visions — his dream-like trances — occurred on his walks, even on the half-mile or so trip from his lodgings to school, although he usually extended that to a five-mile walk by going around a lake. Around 1800, Wordsworth and his sister Dorothy went for morning and evening walks around the area of their home, with each of those two- and three-hour jaunts being part of their daily routine. Sometimes they did even longer walks, to see friends, for example. Dorothy wrote in an 1804 letter to a friend, "At present he is walking and has been out of doors these two hours though it has rained heavily all morning. In wet weather he takes out an umbrella; chooses the most sheltered spot, and there walks backwards and forwards and though the length of his walk be sometimes a quarter or half a mile, he is as fast bound within the chosen limits as if by prison walls. He generally composes his verses out of doors and while he is so engaged he seldom knows how the time slips or hardly whether it is rain or fair." In the fall of 1831, when he was over 60, Wordsworth usually managed to walk 20 miles a day. Dorothy often went on those long walks with her brother and in 1828, at age 56; she said she could still walk 15 miles as briskly as ever. At the age of 79, the writer was still going out and taking little walks in his home area and to visit friends, although the distances of such sojourns were greatly diminished.[11]

William Hazlitt (1778–1830) remarked, "I like to go by myself. Nature is company enough for me. I cannot see the wit of walking and talking at the same time." In an 1822 essay, Hazlitt exclaimed, "Give me the clear blue sky over my head, and the green turf beneath my feet, a winding road before me and a three hours' march to dinner — and then to thinking!" Immanuel Kant (1724–1804), founder of the transcendental school of philosophy, walked for one hour every afternoon.[12] Jane Austen (1775–1817) also loved long walks. While living in Bath in 1801, she went for a long and energetic walk with a neighbor, Mrs. Chamberlayne. Of that walk she wrote, "I could with difficulty keep pace with her — yet would not flinch for the world." A few days later they went walking again together and Austen managed to keep up with her. In Bath as visitors in the period 1804–1805, were the Reverend Samuel Cooke and his wife Cassandra, cousin to Jane's mother. Their daughter Mary and son George went with Austen on long walks. In the period 1809, the Austen sisters usually went for long walks, after lunch, sometimes into a nearby town for shopping, sometimes to visit people.[13]

Sir Walter Scott (1771–1832) took walks of 20 to 30 miles over the hills of his native land, while Samuel Taylor Coleridge (1772–1834) did a daily 10-mile sojourn. Often he walked alone and was also partial to night walking. Around 1795, walking tours were becoming a new fashion, with young men from the universities dressed as tramps and wandering through the countryside, staying at local inns, talking enthusiastically with "the common people," hill climbing, communing with nature, and so forth. Wordsworth had crossed the Alps into Italy, Bowles had wandered through Wales and Germany, and Coleridge that year planned his own "pedestrian scheme" through the Wye Valley and up into Wales. His walking companion was fellow undergraduate Joseph Hucks. That was the first of Coleridge's many epic walks. During one part of that 1795 trip they covered over 500 miles in just over one month. On the way, he bought the first of many notebooks because, he said, "as I journey onward, I ever and anon pluck the wild Flowers of Poesy."[14]

Percy B. Shelley (1792–1822) was a cross-country walker who covered mile after mile. William Gladstone (1809–1898) was said to have often walked the streets of London at night. Abraham Lincoln was another American president who was a great walker. A strong proponent of the activity was Charles Dickens (1812–1870), who once remarked, "The sum of the whole is this; walk and be happy; walk and be healthy. The best way to lengthen our days is to walk steadily and with a purpose. The wandering man knows of certain ancients, far gone in years, who have staved off infirmities and dissolution by earnest walking — hale fellows, close upon ninety, but brisk as boys." He was prone to walk the streets of London at night for inspiration. On his triumphal tour of North America in 1842 — although he was in the habit of walking "through and through" the towns he visited — in New York he broke that rule and hired a cab. He did that because there were still many pigs running loose in New York.[15]

Dickens took long walks by which he believed he rested from his mental labors; he put in seven or eight miles at a time at a fast pace. When angry or annoyed or upset he often turned to walking and, said his biographer Edgar Johnson, "he struggled furiously to subdue these fits of spleen, striding fiercely for hours along the cliffs with a seething intensity that disturbed both his work and his rest." In the writing of his *Christmas Carol*, explained Johnson, he "wept and laughed, and wept again, and excited himself in a most extraordinary manner in the composition; and thinking whereof he walked about the black streets of London fifteen and twenty miles many a night when all sober folks had gone to bed." Often, if he had guests at home, he suggested a walk, "but of those who had walked with him before only the bravest dared face the gruelling ordeal again," because, whenever he walked, "Dickens maintained a relentless pace of four miles an hour, swinging his blackthorn stick and talking cheerfully all the way." A "portly" American, Edward Yates, who started out with Dickens and others on one of his walks, had to drop out along the way. He was not the only one to fail to finish a walk with the author. When the group finished their trek that day Dickens saluted those who kept up with him and finished the walk: "Well done! Twelve miles in three hours." That was in the period 1865 to 1870. During that same period, while in America, Dickens took a walk of five miles in the snow at a pace of four and a half miles per hour, from which his two walking companions returned exhausted.[16]

Reporter Hildegarde Hawthorne declared in 1926 that English writer George Meredith (1828–1909) "stands as the finest walker of them all. He loved to walk; walking was to him an essential part of living, bound up with his daily existence." When he was in his 20s he regularly went for walks of 30 to 40 miles a day, according to his biographer Robert Sencourt. He viewed hard exercise as an essential element of a boy's life and as critical in a man's. Meredith urged the joys of the Spartan life for schoolboys. For years while he was in his 20s he walked back and forth over the downs of Epsom. In the days when walking was itself a sport, he was an eager walker; in the days of walking matches—from London to Dover or Canterbury and back—he walked part of the road with the champions. Sencourt said such men were heroes to Meredith. "A man should sweat once a day—then he will have a clear brain," said Meredith.[17]

In the 1860s, one of Meredith's walking companions was William Hardman. And, said Sencourt, "They had in these long rambles a sort of ecstasy as they breathed in the scent of Surrey pinewoods, or watched in autumn the changing tints in elms and beeches. Returning to the cottage, they would eat a plain meal of bread with jam, or honey, and start out again." Like Dickens, Meredith always walked at a fast pace, he never sauntered. In the words of his biographer, "Such walks were Meredith's inspiration: they are central in his history; he was at the same time giving hard exercise to brain and flesh and spirit...." Once, in 1861, he went for a long trek with Frederick Maxse and Thomas Wyse, but Meredith, who could easily walk 30 miles on a hot summer day, grumbled about the lack of endurance shown by Wyse: "He couldn't walk in the sun; he wouldn't walk after its setting; the rain he shunned as if he had been dogbitten — in fact he was a double knapsack on my back." At the age of 50, his love of exercise was as strong and as passionate as ever, although as the years went by his walks became shorter in length. From his walks and his observation of nature, said Sencourt, "he found the inspiration for both his novels and his poems and" felt he "must have occasional movement to be fecund." A rapid walker, wrote Meredith in his *The Egoist*, "poetically minded, gathers multitudes of images on his way." Around 1879 he was one of about 20 men who met every Sunday from October to June to take long Sunday walks.[18]

Ralph Waldo Emerson (1803–1882) once said that "Walking has the best value as gymnastics of the mind." And that philosophic writer believed that "no pursuit has more breath of immortality to it." To treat a liver ailment he once walked 1,000 miles in 90 days around his garden. Another Emerson observation was, "'Tis the best of humanity that goes out to walk."[19]

Perhaps one of the best-known of the famous walkers from the past was Henry David Thoreau (1817–1862) who regarded his daily excursions around Walden Pond as essential for maintaining his mental equilibrium. "I think I cannot preserve my health and spirits unless I spend four hours a day at least — and it is commonly more than that — sauntering through the woods and over the hills and fields, absolutely free from all worldly engagements," he said. With a slow, sauntering style of walking wherein he thought and contemplated and isolated himself from people and urban areas, Thoreau (and others) were opposite to the pound-the-city-streets-rapidly style adopted by Dickens (and others).[20]

To emphasize the difference, Thoreau remarked, "The walking of which I speak has nothing in it akin to exercise as the winging of dumbbells or chairs, but is itself the enterprise and adventure of the day. If you would get exercise, go in search of the springs of life." Thoreau thought of the connection between walking and human well-being in general terms. When he decided to go for a walk, he said, "I seek the darkest woods, the thickest and most interminable and, to the citizen, most dismal swamp." Another time he remarked, "I have met with but one or two persons in the course of my life who understood the art of Walking, that is, of taking walks—who had a genius so to speak, for sauntering."[21]

When he wrote about the isolation of his home, in the period 1842 to 1843, Thoreau also mentioned how many miles he regularly covered: "I can easily walk ten, fifteen, twenty, any number of miles, commencing at my own door, without going by any house, without crossing a road except where the fox and the mink do." On occasion, he walked, he said, "as one possessing the advantages of human culture, fresh from the society of men, but turned loose into the woods, the only man in nature, walking and meditating to a great extent as if man and his customs were not." His friend and sometime walking companion Ellery Channing remarked around 1850, "His habit was to go abroad a portion of each day, to field or woods on the Concord River.... During many years he used the afternoon for walking, and usually set forth about half-past two, returning at half-past five." As a great lover of solitude, he mostly went for walks alone but not always. Thoreau once told Channing he carried no stick with him on his sojourns because even that would be too much company. His friend, Ralph Emerson, observed that Thoreau was a good swimmer, runner, skater, and boatman, and would probably outwalk most countrymen on a day's journey.[22] Much of the thoughts and ideas Thoreau had on walking, some of which are noted above, appeared in one of the philosopher's most celebrated essays, "The Joy of Walking." Although he delivered it repeatedly in the decade of the 1850s it was not published until a month after his death.[23]

Matthew Arnold (1822–1888) was another whose name recurred in accounts as one of the more prominent pedestrians, as well as Robert Louis Stevenson (1850–1894). In a short work entitled "Walking Tours," Stevenson discussed his personal preference for walking style; "I do not approve of leaping and running. Both of these hurry the respiration; they both shake up the brain out of its glorious open-air confusion, and they break the pace. Uneven walking is not so agreeable to the body, and it distracts and irritates the mind. Whereas, once you have fallen into an equable stride, it requires no conscious thought from you to keep it up." If you walked alone, he pointed out, you entered into "the great fellowship of the Open Road. Alone, you have plenty of time for meditation, and, hungry at the end of the day's journey for companionship, you are in a receptive mood for those brief but priceless meetings which only trampers know."[24]

For his 700-mile walk from Toul, in northeastern France, to Rome, the contents of Hilaire Belloc's (1870–1953) pack consisted of "a large piece of bread, half a pound of smoked ham, a sketch book, two Nationalist papers, a quart of the wine of Brule, a needle, some thread and a flute."[25]

Friedrich Wilhelm Nietzsche (1844–1900) remarked, "A sedentary life is the real sin against the Holy Spirit. Only those thoughts that come by walking have any value." Walking as a concept and activity wound its way in and out of his theory of "superman" and his doctrine of the perfectibility of man through forcible self-assertion. He used a steep footpath leading to the isolated village of Eze to walk along to help him create *Thus Spake Zarathustra*. At the end of that footpath, near the gate to Eze, was a plaque containing some of Nietzsche's words, "... during the difficult ascent — the creative inspiration was strongest in me, when my muscles were working the hardest."[26]

John Ruskin (1819–1900) walked six miles a day; it was part of his formula, which entailed getting up at six, walking six miles and then working for six hours. Gustave Flaubert (1821–1880), before he sat down to do his writing, took long walks to relax his breathing and allow his creativity to flow. During the day he would often refresh himself with shorter walks.[27] George Macauley Trevelyan (1876–1962), noted English historian and essayist, once said, "I have two doctors, my left leg and my right. When my body and mind are out of gear (and those twin parts of me live at such close quarters that the one always catches melancholy from the other) I know that I shall have only to call in my doctors and I shall be well again." On another occasion Trevelyan commented, "I never knew a man go for an honest day's walk for whatever distance, great or small ... and not have his reward in the repossession of his own soul."[28]

In more recent times — the 20th century — the number of famous people known for walking has dramatically decreased, and relative to the distances covered by people prior to the 20th century, has vanished altogether. At the beginning of February 1908, it was revealed that General J. Franklin Bell, chief of the U.S. General Staff, had interested President Theodore Roosevelt in William Muldoon's 15-mile test on foot, which was apparently a minor fad of the time. The president was said to have exhibited great curiosity as to the Muldoon system of "fitting fat statesmen" for the Washington dinner season since Secretary Root and General Bell took the course at White Plains. Somewhat sceptically, Roosevelt agreed to try the system wherein the Muldoon test was eight miles at a walk and seven miles at a trot, presumably one right after the other. Bell went over the course easily. Roosevelt completed the course, but not easily. At a dinner two days later, President Roosevelt admitted he had lost all appetite for the Muldoon tests.[29]

More enthusiastic about the activity was William J. Gaynor, mayor of New York City in June 1911, when he authored an article in praise of walking. Since there was said to be great public interest in the mayor's pedestrianism the magazine, *The Independent* got Gaynor to explain himself to its readers. During the 16 years he had been a justice of the Supreme

Court, said Gaynor, "I made it a rule to walk from five to seven miles a day. I did this to keep myself in health.... When I became Mayor I simply continued my walking." He added, "I walk for health, and also for the joy of walking. I have for many years done my principal work while walking. As a judge I framed my decisions and opinions in my mind while walking. I can think best while walking, and then I can come in and sit down and write offhand the whole subject." With respect to journalists, observed Gaynor, "My walking seemed to astonish them." He preferred to walk alone and to think and believed, "There is a feeling of independence and freedom when you are walking and your blood warms up and flows freely, and your body becomes purified." For those people who would not walk, Gaynor advised them to ride a bicycle.[30]

Arts writer and critic J. Brooks Atkinson said in 1923 that he had long taken Sunday morning walks. One reason he picked that time went back to his youth, when he was looking for reasons to avoid attending church. For another, he did not like the type of crowd one found out walking on Sunday afternoons, "For such as we there is no virtue in walking on Sunday afternoons, when the roads are filled with mothers and fathers pushing baby carriages, amorous fellows and girls, and tough adolescents who smoke cigarettes and foul the air with blasphemy — all dressed, according to the familiar phrase, in their Sunday best. Middle class promenading!" Atkinson concluded, "Walking in the serenity of that morning puts aside the petty brawls of the world more effectively than the preacher who feels that he must discuss them in a moral tone. Six days devoted to the handling of phases, of which life is largely composed, requires at least one of feeling the solid earth under foot."[31]

When Viscount Grey of Fallodon gave advice to the boys of Epsom College in England in 1926, he counselled them to "Keep your legs." He warned them against giving up walking in favor of riding bicycles and doubted whether all the modern mechanical contrivances were beneficial. According to Grey, even a middle-aged man was better off walking 20 miles a day than riding 50 on a bicycle.[32] American actor, playwright, and producer George M. Cohan (1878–1942) recommended a walk to banish dejection and despair. "You never heard of anyone," he said, "doing away with himself after a long walk."[33] Reporter J. M. Flagler argued in 1958 that British writers had been among the foremost exponents of walking, and concluded that may have been the reason the British people were the world's most avid pleasure walkers. In England, the pressures to get out and walk were so great that contrarian Max Beerbohm was once moved publicly to denounce the excesses of what he called "walk-mongers." In his essay, "Going Out for a Walk," he declared, "It is a fact that not once in all my life have I gone out for a walk. I have been taken out for walks; but that is another matter."[34]

When Thomas Wolfe was finished writing for the day, said his biographer Elizabeth Nowell, he was keyed up and "he would stride like a wild, disheveled giant through the streets of Brooklyn." In the 1920s, when he and his editor, Maxwell Perkins, were working together on *Look Homeward, Angel*, Perkins would take Wolfe out to dinner "and go with him on his habitual long walks, heroically keeping up with Wolfe's tremendous strides and inexhaustible supply of energy." Never could Wolfe relax enough to go to bed until dawn. He wrote that at the end of a day of creative writing his mind remained so active "I was unable to sleep, unable to subdue the tumult of these creative energies, and as a result of this condition, for three years I prowled the streets, explored the swarming web of the million-footed city and came to know it as I had never done before." From Brooklyn he often walked for miles on end, sometimes ending up far out in the Bronx. Wolfe wrote of his habit of walking, in 1933, after a "furious" day of writing, "and then night again, a frenzied prowling of a thousand streets, and so to bed and sleepless sleep again, the nightmare pageantry to which my consciousness lay chained a spectator."[35]

While he was in Washington, D.C., President Harry S. Truman used to get up at 5:30 a.m., read all the newspapers and then take his half-hour constitutional. By 1961, when he was 78, he continued that practice in whatever city he was in and walked at a pace of 120 steps to the minute (brisk). Asked by reporters why he took his famous early morning stroll, Truman replied, "I believe it will make me live longer." Truman walked early in the morning to minimize interference, that is, later in the morning he was likely to encounter too many pedestrians to maintain his desired pace.[36]

In the mid 1980s, U.S. Senator William Proxmire (D — Wisc.) walked the five miles from his office to his home, while Henry Kissinger, since his bypass operation, walked four miles a day on his doctor's orders. Supreme Court Justice William O. Douglas was known to be a prominent walker.[37] About the same time, Steve Reeves, a former Mr. Universe and the Arnold Schwarzenegger of the Eisenhower era, had been a walking evangelist for 10 years and insisted "walking is not for sissies." Reeves began walking with weights around 1977 — after a series of jogging injuries, working up to a total of 40 pounds (20 percent of his body weight) wrapped around his waist and ankles and held in his hands. Reeves called it powerwalking and in 1982 wrote a book with that title. In 1987 Reeves powerwalked three times a week, 45 minutes each time. That same year, noted actor Helen Hays had been an avid walker for nearly all of her 87 years, a fact that was a source of constant anxiety for her stage managers. "I've always taken walks between rehearsals and performances of plays I've acted in," she explained. "The stage managers have always been nervous that I wouldn't get back in time for my performances." Hays strongly believed that walking was the best exercise of all. Michael Dukakis, a former governor of Massachusetts and presidential candidate, began running back in high school and did not stop until he reached the age of 50 (in 1984), when his body started to complain. So Dukakis switched to fitness walking with three-pound weights. He said he came back to his hotel at 10:30 p.m. after a 16-hour campaign day, picked up his three-pound weights and went out for a fitness walk. "Sometimes it's to think, other times it's just to clear my head, and still other times it's just a chance to get back to nature with a walk through the park," Dukakis explained.[38]

One person *not* impressed with walking in recent times was actor Peter O'Toole. Around 2000, O'Toole quipped, "The only exercise I take is walking behind the coffins of friends who took exercise."[39]

As the 20th century began, and unfolded, it became apparent to observers that the number of people who walked and the distance they covered on foot were shrinking drastically. It seemed, as the popular phrase had it, that nobody walked anymore.

# 3
# Nobody Walks

"*Walking bats a low average today as an avocation.*"
Hildegarde Hawthorne, 1926.

"*Walking is on the way out.*"
*Times* (London) editorial, 1958.

"*Not walking to school is just one example of how walking has largely vanished as a normal, routine part of life.*"
Mark Bricklin, 1995.

Although the idea that nobody walked anymore was expressed mainly in the 20th century, it occasionally surfaced earlier. In 1798 Louis Philippe of France, the Duc d'Orleans, wrote, "An American will never walk if he can ride."[1] New York City Mayor William Gaynor thought in 1911 that the English were the best walkers, but in New York "people are afraid to walk a mile. The greatest rapid transit facilities in the world right here.... Wherever you are here in the city of New York you have a street car at your elbow. The result is that everybody rides and almost nobody walks. This is harmful." Gaynor added, "I drove for years. Out of that I really got nothing. The street car I always abominated." As he walked over the Brooklyn bridge every night and saw the cars traveling along "packed with anemic young men and women, some of them with cigarets, I cannot help pitying them. Why do they not get out and walk and make their bodies ruddy and healthy?" According to the mayor some of the people in the cars looked out their windows "and point at me as though I was a curiosity because I walk. I think they are curiosities because they ride and injure themselves with the foul air of the cars."[2]

Writing in *Saturday Night* in 1912, a journalist lamented the lost art of walking and began his article cynically: "Of course, people still walk. That is, they shuffle along on their own pins from the door to the street-car or the taxi-cab.... They may walk several blocks from shop to shop... But real walking ... is as extinct as the dodo." Answering his own question as to where the walkers went he remarked that some of them had died, "And the rest of them take a street-car down to the office in the morning, and drive out with the family on Sunday in an automobile. And they have become red-faced and fat and their legs are grown wondrous thick." Blamed in this account for the demise of walking was the automobile.[3]

A 1924 account in *The Forum* declared there were two schools with respect to locomotion; one was to never admit the possibility of walking while the second was to state walking was perfect freedom. "The second [school] is perpetually on the point of closing its door for lack of patronage," while the first school had a "considerable waiting-list," concluded the story.[4]

Writing in 1925, Edmund Lester Pearson bemoaned the fact he lived in a city "where nobody walks." That was because hundreds of thousands of people in that city went from railway to street car, from ferry to subway, from elevated line to bus, from subway to taxi. Or cars took them from their front doors to their offices and back again. Additionally, "There are lifts and moving stairways to help them up or down, and every contrivance to promote the atrophy of the human leg. They say they haven't time to walk — and wait fifteen minutes for a bus to carry them an eighth of a mile. They pretend that they are rushed, very busy, very energetic; the fact is, they are lazy. A few quaint persons — boys, chiefly — ride bicycles." Pearson continued his lament by remarking, "They will wait and crowd into a jammed and stuffy elevator rather than walk up even 1 flight of stairs. And they will wait with the same patience rather than walk down a flight or two."[5]

One year later journalist Hildegarde Hawthorne noted that "Walking bats a low average today as an avocation," despite the fact that a walker was "one of the happiest of God's creatures. He's free! No machinery intervenes between him and his enjoyment." She thought that one of the reasons walking was not more popular "is its simplicity. What's the fun of an easy thing?"[6]

An editorial in the *New York Times* in 1928 mentioned area pioneer Ezra Meeker who had just celebrated his 97th birthday and, on the whole, found the world to be slowly and steadily improving in all respects, except one: "There are too many expert mechanical devices now to help people escape walking." Examples given were trains, boats, cars, and airplanes. That editorial generated some response and in one of the letters to the editor in reply, the writer argued that the pedestrian had vanished mainly due to safety concerns. He explained he was constantly apprehensive "whenever I essay to walk a few blocks, and am exposed at every crossing, despite the greatest possible care on my part, to the recklessly contemptuous practices of the average auto driver who grins derisively when one is successful in escaping his assaults by a hair's breath."[7]

Mary Magennis asserted, in 1931, "But to dyed-in-the-wool walk-lovers the car has proved a calamity ... because unless we be strong as steel, our lazy and baser natures yield to the temptation of time-saving when a ride is offered us." She rued the fact "You could walk along the road many a day at any hour you chose and not meet a soul walking, be the day ever so fine."[8]

Another *New York Times* editor returned to the subject of walking in 1942, when he observed that probably no form of exercise was the subject of as much hypocrisy as was walking. That was because thousands of people stated every day, emphatically and without batting an eye, that they loved to walk, "yet don't mean a syllable of it." He added that, for a great many people, walking was all right if there was a worthwhile destination such as a friend's house, a public library, or a neighborhood cinema, "but the aimless ramble had best be read about to be enjoyed thoroughly."[9]

When American family doctors assembled at the 7th annual meeting of the American Academy of General Practice in the spring of 1955, the lack of walking was decried. Covering that convention, reporter Gladwin Hill declared that young people were forgetting how to walk: "They jump into a car to go a block. The trend has already produced conspicuous changes in their physiques." An editorial in the magazine *America*, prompted by that convention, urged more walking for everybody, but especially for young people.[10] When *Harper's Magazine* ran a piece on pedestrians in 1957, it cited a recent *Vogue* article wherein were published a series of interviews with doctors on the subject of losing weight. Asked how effective walking was as an exercise to lose weight, one doctor replied, "Wonderful, but walking has just about disappeared as a public institution." In that same year reporter Howard O'Hagan remarked in Canada's national news magazine, *Maclean's*, that the average Canadian walked a bit less than two miles a day and "walking is not only avoided, as though it were God's punishment to man in this place below, but is even looked down upon."[11]

Writing in *American Mercury*, also in 1957, journalist Murray T. Pringle declared that over the years the average American had become almost totally dependent upon mechanical transportation. Foot experts, he continued, had pointed out "that no American generation has walked less than the present one, or has paid less heed to Thomas Jefferson's dictum that 'Of all exercises, walking is the best.'"[12] One year later J. M. Flagler, in the *New Yorker*, looked back with nostalgia to the time of Edward Weston and all the long-distance walking that took place then in America, and to all the media coverage it received. By contrast, he lamented, "Nowadays, though, distance, endurance, and speed walking are all but lost arts in America." Nobody walks, he stated.[13]

Around the same time, that same sentiment — that nobody walked — was expressed in Europe. An editorial in the *Times* (London) explained that martlets had the proud distinction of appearing without feet on heraldic shields because, as one story went, "they walked them clean off as pilgrims to Jerusalem." It was a lead-in before the editor declared that "walking is on the way out" — for people in both town and country alike. Walking feats were still being accomplished, he said, like breaking the record for walking from Oxford to Cambridge, "But, for everyday purposes, a wait in a queue or a squash in a Tube is preferred to what the doctors so often tell us is the healthiest exercise." Earlier generations, he added, "less dependent on wheels, thought nothing of walking for miles to and from work."[14]

Listing some of the reasons for the demise of walking, in 1961, Theodore Irwin remarked, "Golf carts ... that transport lazy men from tee to tee, drive-in churches, banks and movies make walking nonessential. The other day I noticed a neighbour get into her car to drop a letter into a mailbox only a few hundred steps away." Concluded Irwin, "The trouble with most Americans is that walking is becoming a forgotten sport and a lost art. People would rather jam themselves into crowded buses than ambulate a dozen blocks. Some people even rent electric carts to take them around a golf course."[15]

Commenting on the situation in 1965, Robert Thomas Allen wrote, "When I was a kid, walking was not only the accepted way to move from place to place, but a sign of health, sound values and vitality. Driving a few blocks to shop was an indication of decadence."[16]

George O'Connell declared in the *New York Times* in 1980: "Nobody walks anymore." He said President Jimmy Carter — America was then experiencing a sharp increase in the price of gasoline due to a supposed worldwide shortage — had suggested that if each American family would use one less gallon of gasoline each week, the shortages would disappear. Since the average car got 18 miles to the gallon, more than five billion gallons of gasoline would be conserved annually, computed O'Connell, if each family in America would walk, rather than drive, just two and a half miles a day. And walking would provide other benefits, too, he argued: "It stimulates the circulation, improves muscle tone, unclutters the mind and is vastly superior to diets or diet pills as a way to shed flab."[17] During an

11-day transit strike in New York City in April 1980, millions of New Yorkers were said to have rediscovered a long-ignored activity — walking. However, said reporter Jane Brody, "Unfortunately, when the strike ended, nearly all returned to their motor-driven methods of getting around."[18]

Taking an oddly different stance on the idea that nobody walked anymore was Susanna Levin, in 1987, when the activity was in the midst of having been rediscovered, at least briefly, and was enjoying its then status of being a fairly hot fad. Levin argued that whether or not people bought the idea that walking was exercise, "walking is no trend; it will never be 'out' — imagine someone saying 'Oh, nobody walks anymore.'"[19]

Journalist Mark Bricklin remarked in 1995 that few children walked to school anymore. Back in 1930, he reported, only seven percent of school children got bussed to school. By 1948 the percentage was still below 25. But in 1995, it was 53 percent, and about half of the rest had chauffeurs — their parents. "Not walking to school is just one example of how walking has largely vanished as a normal, routine part of life," stated Bricklin.[20]

Author Bill Bryson and his wife returned to live in the U.S. after 20 years of residence in the United Kingdom. He wanted to live in a town small enough that they could walk to the business district, so the couple settled on Hanover, New Hampshire, in part because of its compactness. Bryson wrote in 2001 that, "It is, in short, an agreeable place to go about one's business on foot, and yet as far as I can tell, virtually no one does."[21] Despite all such sentiments, some walking did take place. Long-distance walking, which disappeared almost entirely in America by around the time of World War I, was revived in various ways from time to time after that date but was always a fairly peripheral part of walking after its fade-out in the early 1900s.

# 4
# Long Distance Walking

> *"It seems to me an extraordinary example of human contradictoriness to go any great distance on foot when it is possible to go by train or by motor-car.... It is a reversion to savagery and a foolish pretence that the twentieth century does not exist."*
> New Statesman, 1923.

Examples of long walks undertaken in the early years of the 20th century included one taken by T. J. McAughey in the summer of 1908. The assistant secretary of the Toronto Young Men's Christian Association (YMCA) left that city on July 27 with a message from the mayor of Toronto to the mayor of New York City. McAughey arrived in Ossining, New York on August 8 and in New York City on August 10. Almost a year later, Jack Williams, a reporter from Philadelphia had reached Chicago on his way walking from Philadelphia to Seattle, a distance of 3,800 miles. On May 22, 1909, Williams walked from Laporte, Indiana to Chicago, some 59 miles.[1]

An example of the lies and exaggerations that began to plague the activity, and presumably contributed to its demise, was apparent in a story in the *New York Times* on May 8, 1911. That story was published on page one and was presented by the newspaper of record without comment and in an uncritical manner. Julius Rath of St. Louis was said to have started distance walking in 1897 when he was 14 years old. Initially, he was started off by the St. Louis Club, with whom he had struck a deal whereby he would win $30,000 from the organization if he walked 500,000 miles by 1915. Reportedly he then had 250 books, each of which was full of testimonials from mayors, governors, assorted dignitaries, and so forth, whom he had encountered on his walking tour. Rath's mileage covered by May 1911 was said to be 475,000. To accomplish that total in roughly 13 years,

Rath would have to have walked 36,538 miles per year, or 100 miles a day on all 365 days of each year for all 13 years. Such a feat was, of course, impossible.[2]

William Cromie and nine students from the University of Pennsylvania walked from Philadelphia to New York City, a distance of 105 miles, in three days back in 1911. Each of the students testified to the fact that he felt better after the walk than before; that, instead of losing energy, he had increased vigor, stated Cromie. Two years earlier a walking club was started among students of the University of Pennsylvania, a club which had over 300 members enrolled in 1911. During the college term, walks were taken on Saturdays to places of interest, and culminated in a long walk during the Easter holidays. Many colleges had clubs of that nature, said Cromie, some of which gave credit for walking in lieu of the physical training otherwise required of the students.[3]

At the age of 70, Edward Weston was still getting lots of daily publicity in 1909 as he made his way across America that summer, in his quest to walk across America in 100 days—Sundays excepted—a distance of about 3,900 miles. Weston had, for example, his own byline in the pieces appearing in the *New York Times*. In those regularly appearing pieces he gave a day-by-day account of his progress and his doings.[4]

Arriving in San Francisco in July of that year Weston missed his self-imposed 100-day time limit, taking 105 days to complete the journey and averaging 37 miles a day. In the opinion of a commentator writing in the *Nation*, that long walk "is an effective protest against the present-day craving for speed in locomotion."[5]

When he was 83, Weston walked from Buffalo, New York, to New York City, a distance of 500 miles. At the age of 87, he was still walking and was listed as the author of an article in a *Saturday Evening Post* issue that year wherein he gave vague and largely meaningless advice for others who wished to do distance walking, such as to wear comfortable shoes and to eat properly. Mostly, the lengthy article described some of his longer sojourns. At almost the same time, an editorial in the *New York Times* discussed Weston and his accomplishments at length. Distance walking by then had all but disappeared from the scene. However, Weston and his past exploits still held superstar status and commanded a certain amount of media attention.[6]

Weston wrote in 1926 that walking was "like a perfect massage. It will ease and relax the muscles. But unlike massage it will also strengthen them." During the latter part of the 19th century, when walking competitions aroused wide interest and inspired high stakes, Weston dominated the sport. He once wrote that "It was my purpose to prove that walking ...

kept a man always in condition without overtraining; that if he took care of himself, ate sensibly and avoided strains, he would actually improve with age and never go stale." As the result of a bet in 1861, the 22-year-old Weston undertook to walk from Boston to Washington within 10 days, to arrive in time for Lincoln's inauguration. Although he missed his deadline by half a day, his effort caught people's attention and the public fancy. Six years later, Weston accepted a challenge from a walking club in Maine to walk from Portland to Chicago, a distance of 1,326 miles within 30 consecutive days (Sundays again excepted) for a purse of $10,000. He told one reporter he wanted to become the "propagandist for pedestrianism," to impress on others the pleasures and beneficial effects of taking exercise in the open air. On that 1867 trip, Weston beat the deadline by one hour and 20 minutes and became a "sensation" overnight. Back in New York he was swamped with invitations to take part in county fairs and weekend walks, and to give lectures and walking exhibitions up and down the East Coast.[7]

Sportswriter Henry Chadwick noted in *Beadle's Dime Handbook of Pedestrianism* that up to the time of the "great" 1867 walking match against time, that was successfully undertaken by Weston, "the art of walking as a healthful exercise had never been considered one of the popular exercises of Americans. It is a well-known fact that where twenty Englishmen can be found who could walk forty miles between sunrise and sunset without any extraordinary fatigue, there are not five Americans who can do a third of the distance without great effort and consequent weakness." Chadwick added that the habit of walking had just been too rare. Reportedly, Weston moved at a speed of five miles an hour "for astonishingly long periods" and could sustain that pace for days and weeks. Weston's fame continued to grow and in 1871 he performed in New York City before a full house at the Empire Rink, where he walked 400 miles in four days, 23 hours, and 32 minutes — about 80 miles per day. For that effort he was paid $1,850 of the gate money, plus $300 in bonuses for breaking lap records. When his fame spread to Europe, Weston journeyed to London in 1876. During his first five weeks in England he walked a total of 1,015 miles with over 200,000 English spectators paying to see him. Weston accepted a multitude of fee-paying speaking engagements.[8]

An example of the scams working their way into distance walking could be found in a *Los Angeles Times* article in 1914, datelined Berlin. Therein it was explained that a way of seeing the world and "living without working"— pretending to be on a walking trip around the world for a mythical wager with an equally mythical club or people — had exhausted its possibilities in Prussia. Authorities there were said to have come to the conclusion that such travelers had become so numerous as to constitute a "public nuisance," and the Minister of the Interior had instructed the police to prevent them from selling postcards with their photographs, announcing lectures, or otherwise "molesting the public," and to discontinue the practice of certifying upon their passports or logbooks that they had passed though this or that town. "If a warning does not suffice to make them move on, they are arrested and punished for vagrancy," added the story.[9]

One person opposed to distance walking was an anonymous author whose work appeared in the *New Statesman* in 1923. Specifically, he attacked long-distance walkers who covered 20 miles or so a day from hotel to hotel on walking tours. "It seems to me an extraordinary example of human contradictoriness to go any great distance on foot when it is possible to go by train or by motor-car," he grumbled. "It would be as reasonable to swim instead of travelling by steamer. It is a reversion to savagery and a foolish pretence that the twentieth century does not exist." All that walking, he added, made them so hungry they lost the finer edge of appetite and thus "take greedily to food that a good-natured woman would not give her Pekinese." Then he blustered, "This, it seems to me, is a brutal form of sport that should no more be encouraged than bullfighting." Not that the author was opposed to walking as an activity; his idea of a walk was anything from three to five miles, or up to seven miles, but "if we are suddenly seized by the desire to go a long way, we either take a train or hire a motor-car." After all, he concluded, the main purpose of a walk was not to go anywhere in particular, but to find a good place to sit down: "This, I think, is the only way in which to see the world. If you make yourself a part of the procession, you cannot see the procession."[10]

Early in 1932, a man was spotted walking backward in Berlin. Upon investigation he turned out to be a Texan said to be attempting to walk backward around the world. The only special equipment he carried was a pair of spectacles with small mirrors on the sides so he could see and avoid obstacles.[11] Then there was Dan O'Leary who died in Los Angeles in the spring of 1933 at the age of 91 and was described as a "world-known walker." Back in 1875, he defeated Edward Weston in a six-day race at Chicago. O'Leary once said he could walk 500 miles in six days and then did so. On another occasion he beat Weston again in a walking match in England and won a prize of $14,000. Members of the English parliament gave him a dinner with William Gladstone being the chief speaker. However, in 1896 Weston beat O'Leary badly. Throughout much of O'Leary's life, his habits included taking a daily 20-mile walk with a 100-mile sojourn once a year to celebrate his birthday. Reportedly, O'Leary enjoyed excellent health until one year before his death.[12]

Dance marathons enjoyed a certain prominence in the 1930s, but so did walkathons, albeit to a lesser extent. In Minneapolis, Minnesota, in

1933, between 10,000 and 12,000 people jammed an auditorium every night for months to watch one of those spectacles, something described by journalist Meridel Le Sueur as "dramatically inane." According to Le Sueur, perhaps a dozen walkathons with similar attendance figures had been held around the same time in large American cities. Spectators at Minneapolis paid 40 cents for general admission per day, or 70 cents for a reserved ringside seat. That walkathon began with the contestants being allowed 15 minutes of rest each hour, but ended with the rest periods reduced over time to eight minutes an hour, the contestants by then had been on the floor for some two months. Finally the contest was closed by the mayor, with the still remaining contestants—five in number—splitting the meagre prize money of $1,000. Le Sueur remarked, "The mob's excitement, feeding on the tiny bedraggled figures in the arena, is something that at first makes one very sick. Its abandon is awful and shameless." With respect to those spectators, Le Sueur continued, "But they know the nightmare they are watching in all its aspects; they know the suffering of boredom and inertia; they see nothing foreign in the absurdity of a walking individual, dead asleep, being watched by ten thousand people and not knowing it."[13]

Dr. John Huston Finley was the editor in chief of the *New York Times* in 1937 when he was 73 years old. Even then, he walked 10 miles every day, and at least once a year he walked around Manhattan (a distance of 32 miles). "A good walk clears the mind, stimulates thinking," he said. As a tireless proponent of the activity he still gave out medals to faithful walkers—schoolchildren. Finley designed the medal years earlier when he was commissioner of education for the State of New York. On that medal was the figure of a walking boy and the motto "à la Sainte Terre" (to the Holy Earth). "The world of our better selves is most surely reached by walking," he commented.[14]

A 1951 article described Thomas D. Storie of New York and his wife as the world champion city hikers. During the previous 20 years, equipped with a pedometer to keep an accurate account, the Stories had walked city streets to a total of over 15,000 miles. They had walked every street of the five boroughs of New York City and had traversed the main streets of many other cities, including Philadelphia, Pittsburgh, Boston, Baltimore, Chicago, and Denver. It was the Stories' habit to fly or go by train or bus to those cities and then start walking from one end of the city to the other. A year earlier, in 1950, the Stories flew to Bermuda and walked 85 miles out of the total of the miles of streets there.[15] Seven years later, Tom and Catharine Storie and their city walking exploits were profiled again. This account described the Stories as "America's Walkingest Couple." As passionately as Thoreau avoided towns while on his walks, so did the Stories avoid the country. They were dedicated city walkers. Their single day distance record was 19 miles, and they traveled at an average speed of three miles an hour. This 1958 *New Yorker* piece was a very long and affectionate look at the couple.[16]

*Newsweek* reported at the beginning of January 1960 that there was a new fad in the United Kingdom — distance walking. After describing Britain as "a nation of walkers," it reported that a man named Mike Desmond covered the 110 miles from Norwich to London in 30 hours. Then Dr. Barbara Moore, 56, a Russian-born dietician, walked the 110 miles from Birmingham to London in 27.5 hours. Then she walked the 373 miles from Edinburgh to London in seven days — although she was accused of hitching a ride for 14 miles. Then 250 women, representing all auxiliaries of the armed forces, took off at one-minute intervals to walk from Birmingham to London. And thus the fad took hold.[17]

Frank Mercer, 79, owned a St. Albans, England, chronometer factory. After visiting a youth club and watching rock and roll in the summer of 1961, he said that the youth of the day were "just soft sissies." He then challenged his 400 male employees to walk 50 miles in 15 hours for a five pounds Sterling bonus. Thirty-two men accepted the challenge and 16 finished the walk, six of 'em were teenagers. Said Mercer, "I don't retract a single word I said. I am proud of my chaps who completed the walk. But some of them are in their 20s and 30s. Where are the teenagers? Most of them are still lying in bed, I expect. This certainly has not proved me wrong."[18]

What took America by storm in 1963 were the 50-mile (or less) hikes, with the enthusiastic and very public support of President John F. Kennedy. According to one account, it all started when U.S. Marine Commandant David M. Shoup unearthed an old executive order sent out in 1908 by President Theodore Roosevelt that required all Marine Corps officers to be able to walk 50 miles in 20 hours. Shoup sent the memo to Kennedy, who wrote back wondering if the Marines of the day were fit enough to do it. Soon everybody in the country — from children to seniors — was taking one of the old-fashioned distance walks.[19]

To uphold the honor of the Marine Corps Shoup officially designated 34 marines to take a 50-mile hike. All finished the distance within the 20-hour time limit, each carrying a 24-pound pack. Attorney General Robert Kennedy (the president's brother) set off separately with four aides from the Justice Department on his 50-mile jaunt. All four aides had dropped out by the 35-mile mark but Robert went on to finish alone, in a time of 17 hours and 50 minutes. All kinds of groups gave it a try, especially youth organizations. Newspapers, looking for a "bright feature," invariably sent reporters on the road to walk and file first-person accounts. Although the newspapers put their most athletic journalists on the road, reportedly few of them finished. Portly Pierre Salinger (President Kennedy's press secretary) originally promised he would go on a 50-mile walk with newsmen, but then backed out after a bad experience on a six-mile warm-up trip. By then, President Kennedy's Fitness Council had issued warnings of the health dangers of such activity to the unaccustomed and sedentary — even to the point of a heart attack. Said Salinger, "I may be plucky, but I am not stupid."[20]

The whole thing came as a surprise to car-loving Americans who had been subjected for a long time to the seemingly unopposed idea that nobody walked anymore. Everybody tried the 50-mile walk — Boy Scouts, college students, secretaries, newsmen, and politicians, to name but a few. In the midst of the craze, one reporter noted, "a number of physicians were wondering whether the foot bone was even remotely connected to the head bone." U.S. Surgeon General Dr. Luther L. Terry warned, "The 50-mile hike should be built up to gradually and with caution."[21]

Trade publication *Broadcasting* listed in 1963 a great many of those distance jaunts that involved radio and/or television personalities. A few were: a 28-mile walk by Pittsburgh KDKA disk jockey Clark Race, who was accompanied at the start by 5,000 people, (2,000 finished); WFUN Miami, had a 50-mile trip that featured seven of its disk jockeys, marines, soldiers, Boy Scouts, two mailmen, and Mayor Robert King; of the 1,200 who started out on a walk with WAMS, Wilmington, Delaware, disk jockey Dean Tyler, 90 finished the 50-mile distance. Although the 50-mile fad had an intense grip on America, it was very short lived and had been forgotten by the time of President Kennedy's assassination late in 1963. [22]

Philip Shabecoff, a reporter, argued in 1965 that the German people were among the most dedicated and enthusiastic social walkers in the world. They had a wide variety of walking and hiking clubs and a magazine devoted to the activities of those groups. When a Munich newspaper organized a walking contest as a promotion, with no reward on tap except a medal offered to those who completed a 30-mile hike, it did not expect a lot of entrants. However, 8,000 people started and 5,576 completed the distance. Alfred Grieshaber, 78 and said to be as fit and active as men in their 30s, commented, "The secret of my good health is simply walking. I smoke 20 cigarettes a day and drink plenty of wine, but I also walk at least five miles a day."[23]

On occasion, the distance walk was used for political purposes. At the end of March 1970, four men dressed as tramps arrived at Buckingham Palace in London after they had pushed a baby carriage filled with cigarette butts along a 120-mile route from Brighton. The walk was to draw attention to the plight of about 100,000 people down-and-out in Britain.[24] Three months later, about 25,000 people took part in a walk around Britain's coastline in an attempt to raise 100,000 pounds Sterling to rehouse 325 destitute families. For the event, 325 walks averaging 17 miles each had been set up so that participating groups could simultaneously cover the entire 5,500 miles of coastline.[25] One of Britain's best-known distance walkers was John Hillaby (66 years old in 1983), who had by then published four books on his marathon strolls. One, from Land's End to John O'Groats was from one end of Britain to the other. He regularly did stints of 25 miles a day.[26]

Some 739 people went for a 30-kilometer (18.75 miles) walk near Killeen, Texas in 1982. They were on a "volksmarch," a huge group hike that had become popular since it was imported from Germany by U.S. servicemen. Founded in 1977, the American Volksport Association staged only two such events in its first year, but by 1982 it was said that such events were being staged every weekend in 37 states. While the account tried to portray this as some type of new fad catching on in America, that was not the case. Walking was indeed in craze status at this time, but not distance walking.[27]

Marketing became an integral part of the walking craze by the early 1980s and at least one attempt was made to unite marketing with distance walking. In September 1984, Robert Sweetgall embarked on a year-long 11,600-mile trek across the U.S., including Alaska and Hawaii. Along the way, he lectured at school assemblies and community meetings about the dangers of a sedentary lifestyle and the importance of exercise. Sweetgall was participating in a marketing program for Massachusetts-based Rockport Company, a manufacturer of lightweight footwear and walking shoes. Rockport and Gore-Tex Fabrics, a division of Maryland-based W. L. Gorey & Associates, were corporate sponsors of Sweetgall's "Walk for the Health of It" campaign. They were trying to convince Americans to associate exercise with walking. They were also trying to get Americans to associate walking with Rockport shoes and Gore-Tex fitness wear. The brainchild of Carol Cone, president of the Boston marketing firm Cone & Company, the marketing program persuaded a publisher to produce a book for it—*Fitness Walking*—for a September 1985 release by Putnam. "In product marketing you have to enliven the product, you have to make it sexy," explained Cone. But, she added, "how do you make walking sexy? It's like saying, 'Let's do a program on making breathing sexy.'" Cone answered herself: "You can't do it. We take the educational role whenever possible."[28]

The falsification that contributed to the decline in popularity of distance walking in the pre–World War I era could also be found in recent times, even though distance walking was rarely in the news and hardly anybody paid any attention to the activity. It was announced in 1996 that Ffyona Campbell would be removed from the next *Guinness Book of Records* at her own request after admitting that she cheated when she took the title of first woman to walk around the world. In part of the U.S. leg of her supposed 10-year, 19,586 mile jaunt, she hitched rides in her back-up truck that followed along with supplies. She did so because she found she was unable to complete the required 25 miles a day on foot. Thus she rode most of the way in the truck and walked only the last few miles into towns where press conferences were being held. Campbell was listed in the 1997 edition of the book but was to be removed from the 1998 edition.[29]

An examination into the nature of walking, including the types of walks and the philosophy of the activity, along with aspects of women's place in walking were topics that arose once in a while, but almost all such references surfaced long ago. Rarely have such items been mentioned in recent times.

# 5
# The Nature of Walking

*"Pedestrianism is rather a fine art than a means of locomotion.... He who uses his legs is thereby enabled to use his eyes."*
Nation, 1909.

*"The real walker does not move in a herd ..."*
Madge MacBeth, 1914.

*" ... we sense something obsessive and fussy in devoted walkers ... we resist walking because it makes us seem common."*
Peter Steinhart, 1987.

*"Not many women ever learn how to walk ... They manage to get around in an upright position; but not one in ten can walk with ease and grace."*
Good Housekeeping, 1940.

When Arnold Haultain discussed the nature of walking, at very great length in the pages of *Atlantic Monthly* in 1903, he thought that "calm" was a key concept in any discussion of the activity. For him a walk was understood to be something that took place in the country; it was a rural endeavor. Complaining that the game of golf had killed the country walk, Haultain observed that those who believed golf consisted of country walks could not be more wrong, "For mark you, the essence of a country walk is that you shall have no object or aim whatever ... for to start with a determination to cover a certain distance within a specified time is to take not a walk, but a constitutional." The proper frame of mind for a walk, he added, was "that of absolute and secure passivity; an openness to impressions; a giving-up of ourselves to the great and guiding influence of benignant Nature...." Describing walking as a primal instinct as old as Eden, Haultain believed that no mechanical contrivance for locomotion would extirpate the tribe of tourists, of those who walk from love of walking."

Posing a question he thought a practical man might raise, he wondered what pleasure or profit was to be gained from walking, and answered himself by saying, "not the least of the practical blessings incident to a walk is that you are beyond the reach of letters and telegrams and telephones."[1]

Another who believed that a walk should be aimless argued in the pages of the *Spectator* in 1907 that it was a rather "sad affair" when a man going forth for a country walk said that he wanted to have "an object for his walk." It was a sad affair, said the writer, because a walker needed to be open and observant to everything he saw, asking the "why" of everything he saw.[2] A reporter writing in the *New York Times* in 1909 declared that he liked sometimes to set off on a walk totally randomly, with no set direction for the sojourn selected beforehand. As well, he likened the walker to a seer who rose above the constitutional, mainly by keeping his eyes open to his entire environment.[3]

That same year, a writer in the *Nation* observed, "Pedestrianism is rather a fine art than a means of locomotion.... He who uses his legs is thereby enabled to use his eyes. Nature in all moods is the companion of him who walks." Grudgingly allowing that a companion on a walk could be acceptable, he nevertheless cited Hazlitt as having said, "the full flavour of a walking tour is best tasted in solitude." Preserving a peaceful mind was the major purpose of walking and, he added, "The humble mode of walking contains the germ of elemental happiness."[4] A year after that, a contributor to *Atlantic Monthly* asserted that walking "is the primal and the only way to know the world." Although the bicycle permitted the user more speed, it was a "foe to observation while carriages (propelled by horse or motor) destroy all feeling of achievement." A walker walked, he argued, "not to arrive, but to be in the world, to contemplate the same, and to take sufficient leisure for the formation of his judgments." Preferably that leisure was experienced by sitting on a fence during periodic stops from walking.[5]

Country walks were treated favorably again in the pages of *Saturday Night* in 1912, when the contributor remarked there were still a few old-fashioned people who walked to the office every morning, "But when all is said and done, that is not real walking. You can't really walk in city streets. It is not the art of walking, it is nothing but trudging — a far different and much less joyous thing. But it is far and away better than hanging onto a street-car strap." Then he said another pastime confused with walking was more properly called strolling. When one strolled one did not go far and one certainly did not go fast. However, the writer liked "sauntering" [actually, much the same as strolling, being a leisurely ramble], although he did not define it except to call it "the very poetry of walking."[6]

Country walking remained the romantic ideal as the best setting for a walk, at least well along into the 20th century. Elizabeth Onativia wrote a 1929 article in which she expounded on how difficult it was to walk in cities, particularly in New York City. "Pedestrianism in city streets today involves executive ability, planning and foresight, specialized knowledge and concentration," she wrote. A crafty New Yorker, therefore, who was walking for whatever reason "plots his journey like a trip to Europe."[7]

When journalist Madge MacBeth wrote about the topic in general in 1914, she made another point that many early writers made — that walking was an activity best done alone. Noting that walking clubs had disadvantages, MacBeth went on to explain that "the real walker does not move in a herd. She goes alone or accompanied by a very few — congenial spirits, who neither chat nor make such a business of covering ground that they cannot stop to appreciate a bit of landscape."[8]

Late in the 1930s, an article in the *Times* (London) argued that, in England, at least, road walking had disappeared altogether, with another change being the extent to which walking had become organized. At the time, travel agencies then took walkers to the Alps, and Germany, and so forth. Not only did they provide tickets and interpreters, but hotels, planned routes, and guides — "tramping without tears," as it was described. "Inevitably it follows that walking has become a social phenomenon," continued the story. "The solitary walker is a rarity: walking with a single companion is not common." Cited was Arthur Sidgwick who wrote in 1912, "Walking alone is of course on a much lower moral plane than walking in company." The writer of the 1938 article related that he had recently gone on a country walk with some 200 others who showed up. Those people were divided into three walking groups — strenuous, medium, and easy. In the medium group, the pace was set at four miles an hour and "The pace never slackened. There were no pauses to regard the landscape, to listen for the tiny country sounds, or even to take photographs."[9]

Still on the theme of solitary walking, H.F. Ellis declared in 1956, "Walking should be voluntary, uncomplicated, and preferably spur-of-the-moment. This is one of many arguments in favour of walking alone." As the number of people out for a walk together increased, so did the number of difficulties that arose, he explained, because no two people walked at the same pace, and the essence of enjoyable walking was that it should be unregimented. "Freedom from talk is one of the supreme boons of walking alone. Solitude and silence are rare enough to be surprisingly enjoyable once in a while," added Ellis. "Also, the absence of talk makes it much easier to observe, which is another of the pleasures of walking."[10]

As late as 1961, journalist Theodore Irwin repeated some of the same points when he pointed out that many observers contended walking should be a voluntary, uncomplicated, unregimented, preferably spur-of-the-moment idea, and "This is one of many arguments in favour of legging it alone."[11]

One reporter who looked at the nature of walking in great detail was John Kieran, who in 1931, described 12 different types of walks: (1) The Escape, which provided relief from cars and crowded cities; (2) The Constitutional—"an upper-class kind of strolling or walking, probably recommended by an expensive doctor;" (3) The Hike, taken alone or with companions, a trip taken from one point to another with stopover privileges; (4) The Walk for Distance, which was described as not good for the soul as it involved the compiling of distance for the sake of distance; (5) The Daily Jaunt, a trip to and/or from the office to home; (6) The Moonlight Stroll, favored by young people and poets; (7) The Walking Tour, a vacation on foot extending for days, weeks or months; (8) The Winter Walk—"A man comes in from a Winter walk feeling that he has completed an achievement; he has shown his strength"; (9) The Walk Contemplative—advocates of the contemplative walk were Emerson, Wordsworth, and Thoreau; (10) The Walk of Relaxation, short or long, to ease the tedium of the day, the brain rested while the muscles worked; (11) The Companionate Walk, a saunter with friends for the sake of friendship; (12) The Questing Walk, a search for something such as a shrub, bird, or favorite flower.[12]

Kieran thought it would be worthwhile to compile a "walker's anthology of verse," with distinguished contributors to include Tennyson, Wordsworth, Thomson, Shakespeare, Bryant, Keats, and Swinburne. Especially recommended by Kieran were the joys of an invigorating Winter walk, and, he concluded, "Any walk is beneficial, good for body and soul. Apart from the exercise, time spent on such trips clears the mind as the opening of windows clears the air in overcrowded rooms."[13] Also fairly specific was Robert Walker, who published an article in 1934 in praise of walking at night when it was raining. Walker claimed he had walked 30,000 miles in the previous 20 years, of which 6,000 miles were covered at night and 3,000 of those during heavy rains on dark nights. There were times, he remarked, when the mind needed a good cleaning and stimulating tonic, and, "so far as I know, the most wholesome way in some manner involves direct contact with Nature." Walking at night in the rain meant he never ran into anybody—he liked the solitude.[14] Mae Kelly believed, in 1936, that one's mental condition affected one's walk. For example, the person who felt he was a trifle better than his neighbor, or who knew more than someone else, or who had an optimistic outlook on life would express that in his walk. In Kelly's view, the person who felt he was in the way of everyone would walk as if he were trying to remain out of the way.[15]

During the time of World War II, H.L. Brock offered the thought that walkers (excluding hikers and mountain climbers) could be divided into two groups; "There are those who walk to be walking and those who walk to look at things." According to Brock the first type were prone to carry machines that clocked mileage for them and to accumulate large totals, while the other type were really explorers, curious people who loved the scenery of the country such as the woods, fields, and streams.[16]

Speaking in London, England, at a 1937 lunch given to celebrate a new film, *The Health of the Nation,* Sir George Tilly said, "Modern city life with all its contrivances for making legs superfluous, is the enemy of fitness.... The man who doesn't use his legs is on his way to Harley Street [a street best known for its number of doctors' offices]." Nevertheless, a reporter covering that affair cynically speculated that not even two percent of the audience would cover so much as a mile on foot as a result of Tilly's warning. "Walking is natural, but the love of walking is an acquired taste.... How seldom we envy anybody who is walking! What objects of envy, on the other hand, are and have always been those who are sitting in a moving vehicle!" declared the journalist. Admitting he agreed with everything Tilly said and that he did not defend the general "antipathy" to walking, he still went on to argue that walking was too "noble" to be degraded to the level of a medicine bottle. Walking, he felt, should be done for walking's sake or not at all. He did not agree with Hazlitt, R.L. Stevenson, and others, however, who stressed the importance of walking alone. Another whose thoughts on walking he admired was Hippocrates, who once commented, "Walking should be rapid in winter and slow in summer, unless it be a burning heat. Fleshy people should walk faster, thin people slower...."[17]

Journalist Hal Borland argued in 1946 that one could rate a man's curiosity about his world and his fellow man by his walking habits, and that it was not possible to walk without some stimulus to thinking because "The very movement seems to stir the mind into action." All walking, for him, was discovery. While he preferred a walking companion to going solo, it was understood the companion had to be like himself and "the chatterer should be left behind." Borland concluded, "He who walks may see and understand. You can study all America from one hilltop, if your eyes are open and your mind is willing to reach. But first you must walk to that hill."[18]

A 1962 editorial in the *Times* (London) remarked on the fact that many an entrant in the book *Who's Who* had put down "walking" among his recreations. But going one step further was the 70-year-old Lord Birkett, whose choice had been "gentle walking." That prompted the editor to reminisce about the old days of the "great" walkers who regularly covered 30 and 40 miles per day, and to discuss the differences between long and short distance walking. He argued that on a long walk a man might walk himself "into a very pleasant, stupefied state of union with nature, in which he is as happy as a king and about as conscious as a cabbage" and it might be that a man saw more as the distances he covered grew less. "The day comes when he cares no longer about totting up the miles; and he is ready then for gentle walking," concluded the editor.[19]

One of the few writers to deal with the nature and philosophy of walking in the modern era was Peter Steinhart in the pages of *Audubon* in 1987. Americans for the most part were unwilling walkers, he said: "We are not innocent and simple-minded enough to enjoy a walk. It is too slow, too cheap. We crave the astonishing, the exciting, the faraway." For centuries in the Western world, he argued, walking carried the elements of class distinction. As the rich and powerful emerged from an undifferentiated community, they rode in litters, carriages, and yachts to confirm their superior status. Poor people carried the rich and powerful, or deferentially stood aside as they passed. "Today, in the popular view, we sense something obsessive and fussy in devoted walkers," said Steinhart. "Popularly, we resist walking because it makes us seem common." While he found more than 500 associations in America devoted to the automobile, there were only two or three (listed in the *Encyclopedia of Associations* and excluding mountaineering clubs) devoted to walking. As Americans at that time spent four hours a day watching television, Steinhart was moved to say, "We experience life not through the soles of our feet but through the seats of our pants." As a symbol, he argued further, walking was not very potent: "At his inauguration, Jimmy Carter got down from his limousine and walked to the White House. To a few it recalled Gandhi's marches. To others, it was just a small-town stroll." And when Americans did walk, it was often not thought of as a pleasure—dragging the kids through Disneyland, or was seen as a disappointment—walking when the car broke down.[20]

Steinhart observed that all the prodigious walkers were from long ago—when Percy Bysshe Shelley and Mary Wollstonecraft eloped, they walked the first hundred miles—and that they were writers and philosophers rather than bankers and attorneys. That was because walking fed a different part of the mind: "It feeds the intuitive and the imaginative, the perceptive rather than the calculating side of the mind." Another way of putting it, Steinhart declared, was that walking "exercises the senses. The pleasures of walking are the pleasures of having sight, sound, touch, smell and taste all at work together." According to Steinhart, "There is something threatening in walking, because walking is something done by poor people and something that leads us to think and feel in an older, less structured, less disciplined way." He added, "Walking is what we do when we protest. Walking opens up the vents of feelings. It lets us see the world in detail, as it might be, as it ought to be. And that view is dangerous to those who want to rule the world in the narrow grids of profit and votes. That is why artists and writers walk."[21]

Only occasionally were women mentioned as a separate and distinct class of walkers. Winifred Kirkland wrote in 1912 — in a lengthy article in praise of walking, especially in bad weather — that in all the countryside near her home, "I am the only woman who walks." As to the penalty she paid for that uniqueness, Kirkland believed "there is distrust of one who obviously enjoys the zest of her own feet as much as their wives enjoy jogging through life beside a comfortable husband behind a comfortable horse."[22]

In a different article that same year, an unnamed male reporter observed, "When one walks, one walks far and fast and with men. There are a few women one can walk with, but alas, very few." Strolling, though, presented a different story because "When one strolls, one doesn't go far, and one certainly doesn't go fast. And there are a lot of women who make a charming second in a strolling party." But strolling was not walking, "because when you walk, you keep walking, you know."[23]

When Madge MacBeth wrote in 1914 about female walkers, she commented, "For many years, walking, really walking, was a luxury of the few who defied the prevailing fashion which made for languid airs and feminine delicateness, and insisted upon being healthy!" Looking back in time revealed that Chinese women could not be found walking, she argued, nor Japanese women, nor Persian and Turkish harem women and "In France and Italy ladies were not garbed in such a manner as to make walking comfortable." MacBeth wondered why some young woman did not set herself up as a Dog Walker but then concluded by dismissing the idea. "I see now that it is perfectly impractical. Dog Walkers would languish and die as far as their professional careers are concerned: we must have exercise; we cannot hire some one to walk for us, consequently we must air our own dogs."[24]

From the annals of bizarre research came the findings of Dr. John W. Crist of Michigan State College. Based on his study, he reported in 1928 that 54 percent of American women walked with their feet toeing straight ahead, Indian fashion; 41 percent toed out after the old dancing-school pattern; and 5 percent were pigeon-toed. Crist gathered his data by standing on busy street corners during his spare time and unobtrusively recording the walking habits of approximately 11,000 women in various U.S.

cities. He also estimated the age of each subject. Among women in his over-40 group, 75 percent toed out. But that increase was not due to age, he concluded: "Weight is the more important factor. As heaviness increases with age, the feet respond by turning outward. Of the heavily built women over 40, 80 per cent toed out. But only 40 percent of the lightweight women over 40 turned out their toes for fashion."[25]

Mae Kelly observed in 1936, "It is certain that a woman must look to her walk, if she would have ease and grace of movement and retain the slim, symmetrical outlines of youth, long after exercises are shelved and forgotten."[26] Kelly gave women some brief advice in a paragraph or two on how to walk correctly, including the advice that the toes should be pointed straight ahead when a step was taken. However, it was left to *Good Housekeeping* in 1940 to produce a full article on the topic for women, titled straightforwardly, "How to Walk." It was complete with diagrams, because, said the article, "not many women ever learn how to walk. They manage to get around in an upright position; but not one in ten can walk with ease and grace." One tip was for a woman to study her own footprints to see what they revealed. If no sand or snow was available for that purpose the reader was advised to dust her soles with white powder and to walk across the room in her usual fashion. Those footprints should have pointed straight ahead, making a single line one in front of the other, "But if the feet turn out or if there is a double line of prints, you have a lot to learn." Overall advice included "remember to keep your body in line — head up, abdomen flat, pelvis down in back. Hold up your head. Pull up those ribs that want to settle on your hips and give you that thick, middle-aged look. Point your toes straight ahead, and, your knees just grazing each other as you move about." Turning the toes out when walking was said to encourage thick ankles, and if a woman persisted in that habit she could not keep her "good figure." Keeping the legs too far apart while walking resulted in a waddle, which "makes you look old and clumsy, and soon brings on a thick middle section."[27]

Writing in 1962, Jeanne O'Neill described herself as an average suburbanite who only sometimes wanted to go for a walk. Still, she felt she couldn't because it was not socially acceptable. O'Neill admitted she was exaggerating a little; one could walk on a Sunday, the first day of spring, or any time with a dog on a leash, "But if you're young and female and unattached to a baby stroller, walking is dangerously bizarre behaviour."[28]

Rosemary Ellis wrote — in 1986 when walking was in fad status — that some businesswomen who walked to work, or walked during the work day, were concerned that wearing athletic shoes might compromise their professional image. While she thought such behavior was commonplace in

New York City, a more conservative Washington, D.C., like many other cities, was not so accepting. . Patricia Goldman, a walker and vice chair of the National Transportation Safety Board in Washington, D.C., said, "My pet peeve is dress-for-success women who wear Nikes with their business suits. You can buy good flat or low-heeled leather shoes that not only look a lot more professional but also tuck into a briefcase more easily than sneakers." Ellis, however, argued in her article that those businesslike low-heeled or flat shoes did not give enough support for walking.[29]

Walking was something everybody learned to do at around the same time; we just sort of stumbled into it. Prior to World War II, there were very few articles on the topic of how to walk; prior to the 1970s, such articles were almost equally scarce. Then when walking became a big fad in the late 1970s, magazines and books were awash with such advice. Hardly anybody, it seemed, knew how to walk.

# 6
# Instructing the Masses in How to Walk

*"Not many of them [women], as a matter of fact, pay attention to the existing rule of the pavement."*
　　　　　　　　　　　　　　　　Times (London), 1922.
*"Not one man in a hundred knows how to take a walk."*
　　　　　　　　　　　　　　　　Alan Devoe, 1939.
*"The natural way to walk is the wrong way."*
　　　　　　　　　　　　　　　　Pete Martin, 1942.
*"White wool socks are essential for walking any distance."*
　　　　　　　　　　　　　　　　Murray Pringle, 1957.
*"All of the following books on walking contain a large quantity of self-evident material...."*
　　　　　　　　　　　　　　　　Abby Hoffman, 1979.

One area of instruction that was mentioned early but much less later on had to do with what side of the sidewalk people should walk on. They were to walk on the right, at least in North America. Opinion leaders were just as adamant that people walk on the left side of the street in the UK and Australia, for example. One of the earliest such articles appeared in 1924, when M.B. Levick, with tongue somewhat in cheek, outlined the problem of pedestrians walking every which way on the sidewalks. It was a question not of the jaywalker but, thought Levick, of "the master anarchist in all his varieties...." What was needed, he argued, was "a code, a campaign, a walk-on-the-right week...." One benefit from such a campaign was hoped to be that "He who has learned not to jaywalk on the sidewalk would be less apt to jaywalk in the street...."[1]

A letter to the editor of the *New York Times* in 1926 captured some of the sentiment prevalent at the time, when "S.A.M." wondered why we did not insist that pedestrians keep to the right. Since we had white lines on roads for the cars, why not have white lines on the sidewalks and a law to compel walkers to keep to the right. "Keep to the right, properly presented to the people, with information about time-saving and other advantages, ought to become popular," insisted the letter writer. "If it did not the matter is of sufficient importance to warrant legislation."[2] Two years later, Lewis Phillips grumbled in his letter to the editor that it was time liberty was not construed to be license, because "a long-suffering humanity in this crowded city has been subjected to making circles around left-handed walkers." Phillips believed public schools should teach "the proper method of keeping to the right" and then "The school children might bring this home to the elders, with a satisfactory result to follow."[3]

To ease congestion and promote safety, a voluntary method of pedestrian control was put into effect in Detroit, Michigan, during the Christmas holiday season of 1928. Sidewalks, as well as crosswalks at intersections, were marked off in lanes, with large footprints denoting the intended direction of traffic flow. On the sidewalks two fluid traffic lanes were provided, and a third lane alongside the buildings was designated a window-shoppers' lane. Appropriate signs urged the walkers to move appropriately to cross with the traffic, but there was no element of compulsion, as Detroit had no ordinance on pedestrian control. H.M. Gould, newly appointed Detroit traffic engineer, said he hoped "to substitute common sense for compulsion in getting the pedestrian to turn square corners, keep to the right in his own lane and cross streets with the traffic." Apparently the sidewalk markings were placed only on each side of Woodward Avenue for two blocks, from city hall to State Street[4]

Arthur Sproul wrote a pessimistic letter to the *New York Times* noting it was a much tougher job to regulate pedestrians than to regulate motorists. He thought a keep-to-the-right campaign would help a lot, but, while it appeared to be a very simple thing to do and to implement, he believed it would probably never happen.[5]

Three years later another letter writer wanted a plan implemented that began at, say 34th Street for both Broadway and Fifth Avenue, and involved having a white line drawn in the exact center of the sidewalk on both sides of those streets as far north as 59th Street, with pedestrians keeping to the right of the line. However, there would be no objection in crossing the line to enter stores or to window-shop, but otherwise keeping to the right "should be strictly observed."[6]

Decades later, Stewart Beach complained, in 1963 in the pages of *Atlantic Monthly*, about pedestrian drift and various other problems with pedestrians on busy streets, not just a failure to keep to the right. Beach outlined such difficulties as a fast walker trying a pass a wandering slow walker; the forgetful pedestrian who suddenly stopped dead and reversed himself; the two or three abreast who took up the whole sidewalk, and so on.[7]

A couple of decades after that an editorial in the *New York Times* observed that in most places in America traffic moved on the right; "cars do it; boats do it; in most crowded cities people do it. In New York, however, people do not do it." The apparent local rule was described as to be, "Hug the wall." No evidence was presented to show that New Yorkers were unique in that respect nor was any reason given for the New Yorkers' supposed variance.[8]

Reporter Marc Santora wrote a 2002 piece on the poor etiquette displayed by New York pedestrians and indirectly offered some evidence to support the views of the editor who penned his complaint 16 years earlier. Santora also complained about a wide range of poor etiquette practices found in pedestrians, including the sudden stopper, the slowpoke (the "meanderthal"), and "mall" walkers (those who walked three or four abreast and hogged the whole sidewalk). The golden rule for walkers, he said, was to stay to the right. According to this account, Europeans used to driving on the left side of the road had severe problems getting used to New York sidewalks: "They don't know where to go. They are all over the place." In addition, New York was more crowded. In 1991 there were 22,790,000 visitors to New York City; in 2000 there were 37,380,000 visitors. Added to that were Manhattan's 1,537,195 residents and some 800,000 daily commuters.[9]

On the other side of the Atlantic Ocean, back in 1922, authorities in Leicester had spent months trying to encourage the new rule of the sidewalk: "keep to the left." For a start, attention was drawn to the matter by drawing a thick white line down the middle of the pavement with a stenciled request on the sidewalk every now and then saying, "Keep to the left. Safety first." That was followed up with stenciled arrows on the pavement at intervals. However, nothing was very successful.[10]

On July 1, 1922, a new offensive was launched in many districts of London to establish local rules for pedestrian traffic. Several of the metropolitan boroughs had announced their intention of overthrowing the old established rule of the sidewalk, "keep to the right," in favor of the opposite, "keep to the left." The City of London borough was one of the areas not taking part in the initiative. Reason for the change was said to be safety concerns, as it was argued that some street accidents were caused by the existence of a keep-to-the-right custom under which, in certain circumstances, pedestrians walked with their backs to vehicular traffic moving in the same direction, and who in unwary moments stepped off the pavement into the roadway. Mentioned in the article were less than successful campaigns in other cities — Leicester, Glasgow, and Nottingham — to accomplish the same result.[11]

An editorial in the *Times* (London) a couple days later, noting that some areas were changing the rule and others were not, argued that uniformity was desired because, otherwise, pedestrians would be asked to change their positions, theoretically, as they moved from one borough to another, a practice the editor regarded as too confusing. However, he cynically added that a change of rule likely would make little difference in practice "since a large proportion of pedestrians are apparently ignorant, or careless, of the existence of any rule and meander over the footpath at their own sweet will, not only incommoding those who desire to use it for its proper purpose of locomotion, but also putting the community to the heavy expense of widening pavements which in their narrower form would accommodate the traffic were they used in a more orderly manner." In the conclusion, the editor wondered, "Why, we may ask, are children in elementary schools not taught that there is a rule of the footpath which they ought to observe? They learn many things less useful."[12]

Because of that editorial, a woman correspondent wrote to the editor to say the big West End department stores in London did not care about the keep-to-the-left campaign since "they do not believe for a moment that any woman will pay the slightest attention to propaganda when she is looking for bargains." Most of the male heads of those stores, she added, knew that "the conservatism of women is the most difficult thing to break down; that very few women know their left from their right; and that the propaganda of a few weeks will not break down the habits of a lifetime. Not many of them, as a matter of fact, pay attention to the existing rule of the pavement."[13] H.C. Parry wrote to the *Times* (London) in 1928 to state he had received a photo from Adelaide, Australia, showing a white center-line marked on a sidewalk in that city. Parry thought the idea should be extended to busy English towns.[14]

Kristy Sexton wrote about the lack of pedestrian etiquette, in the *Sunday Mail* (Brisbane, Australia), in 2003. She discussed the usual pedestrian faults such as going too slow and stopping suddenly, and declared, "Footpath rage is on the increase because, etiquette experts say, good manners are a thing of the past." Nicole Billante, who recently completed a study on the changing face of social etiquette, said it had become a "free-for-all" on sidewalks. Etiquette expert June Dally-Watkins called for city councils to introduce a keep-to-the-left policy as the number of sidewalk incidents rose. "Staying to the left was once a common courtesy," she said. Under

Australian Road Rule 236, section 2, it was an offense for a pedestrian to "unreasonably obstruct the path of any driver or other pedestrian." In Brisbane's Queen Street Mall [the major downtown shopping area with no cars allowed], pedestrians, declared Sexton, "walk on the left, the right, crisscross, cut each other off and shove each other." Helen McMurray said when she arrived in Brisbane from England 20 years earlier, most city sidewalks had painted lines to enforce the keep-to-the-left custom. "I would like to see that brought back in — people traffic seemed to flow much more smoothly back then," recalled McMurray.[15]

Adding confusion to the keep-to-the-right issue was the 1994 research by John Watson, a cross-national study of walking in public places. First, though, he argued that earlier research showed foot traffic tended to keep right in America and in the UK. Watson's research was conducted in 13 cities in seven nations (England, Denmark, Sweden, Switzerland, Finland, Austria, and Japan) plus the city-state of Singapore. In his study, there were 1,221 observations of 2,442 pedestrians wherein an observation consisted of a solo adult keeping to either the left or right when walking past an oncoming solo adult. Results were that pedestrians in all eight countries kept to the right, with a range of 68 percent to 85 percent for the tendency. Watson concluded that keeping to the right when walking was not linked to the rules that governed vehicular traffic because people in Japan, Singapore and England drove on the left. He thought his results consistent with an earlier researcher's suggestion of a "natural" tendency to keep right when navigating city streets, even though "Such a tendency could even be regarded as maladaptive in Japan, Singapore, and England because it means that pedestrians nearer the curb have their backs to passing motor traffic. Nevertheless, the tendency to keep right is found in those countries."[16]

However, before anybody could go out and keep to the right or the left on the sidewalk, or thumb their nose at the custom, they had to have the basics right, they had to know how to walk. For a long time, experts mostly conceded the point, but as time passed and the populace presumably grew collectively smarter and more sophisticated that consensus changed. More and more the experts decided that people really did not know how to walk. And much of that early advice — as sparse as it was — was concerned with the more general aspects of walking rather than with the narrowly focused, mechanical-approach, instructional pieces that came to dominate later advice. Standing alone as an isolated example from the long-ago past was a 1911 piece that declared the correct way to walk "is to place the heel on the ground first, and have the foot turn slightly outward. The posture of the body is important while walking. The chest should be thrown out strongly, the abdomen drawn in, the chin drawn in toward the chest, the body erect and leaning slightly forward."[17]

Alan Devoe declared in a 1939 piece that it was a "lamentable fact"—not one open to argument—"that not one man in a hundred knows how to take a walk. Walking as an art, as a performance involving subtle spiritual values, is today very nearly extinct." He pointed out that a walk should never have an objective, such as a trip to the supermarket, and that one should just go and walk. That was because a walk must never be a premeditated ritual, but spontaneous. Also, the most important of all requirements for successful walking was the most difficult: "You must learn to expunge from your mind every single one of your usual worriments and vexations." A person who started a walk with a bad worry would find it would only eat at him and get worse, "with the first step you take you must deliberately, by a resolute effort of will, cast off your everyday preoccupations...." Devoe added, "Do not (and there is no more vital walking rule than this) let your attention be arrested by people, instead, open your eyes to the wonders of everyday things—to Nature."[18] More mechanically oriented advice began to appear around the same time. James Hocking celebrated his 85th birthday in 1942 by taking a 55-mile walk. He said a heel and toe stride was necessary, and the feet had to point straight ahead, not to the sides; the body should be carried erect with the arms swinging naturally. Hocking believed that in order to be a "consistent" pedestrian, a person had to do at least 20 miles every week of "vigorous tramping."[19]

Pete Martin observed in 1942 that with America then at war there were 20 percent fewer cars on the road and the situation was expected to get worse, with looming tire and gasoline shortages for civilian purposes. This meant Americans would have to do more walking, speculated Martin, and he worried that the Germans and the Japanese had an edge on the U.S. in leg strength. Encouraged by the state, he related, bands of young Nazis had made a cult of walking, while the Japanese spent a "major portion of their lives squatting or raising themselves up from a squatting position, with the result that they have the strongest, best-developed legs in the world...." We needed more leg power to compete with the enemy, he concluded. For the average man, said Martin, "the natural way to walk is the wrong way. Left to their own devices, men, women and children walk ungracefully and inefficiently [although he did not explain how]. Correct ways to walk must be studied and worked at," advised the reporter. Borrowing from the Boy Scouts of America and from the Office of the Surgeon General of the U.S. Army (both had made a study of walking), Martin offered the usual suggestions and advice, such as toes straight ahead, head held erect, and arms hanging loosely and swinging in time with the stride. "Never saunter," he warned. "Sauntering is the most tiring way to walk." Martin also went on at length to discuss shoes and socks, giving such obvious advice as that the socks should be clean and the shoes must fit.[20]

George Fitzgerald went a little further in 1943, offering classes in walking, partly, at least, because of the war causing more people to become walkers. It was said that thousands of people who had to store their cars as well as others attended Fitzgerald's free weekly evening classes in Brooklyn, New York. After a short film and a lecture, Fitzgerald showed them what was wrong with their walking. First step was to walk in a set of footprints in his classroom. Students were taught to walk with feet close together, toes straight ahead, body erect, and with a springy step. During the day, Fitzgerald and his partner, Harry Palter, operated a large shoe store. Fitzgerald walked to and from work daily, a total of four miles.[21]

A one-page article in the May 1946 issue of *Good Housekeeping* offered mostly photographs but also included a list of dos and don'ts— For example, "Do make the back foot propel you forward by giving a little push-off with it, directing the force against the pelvis. This way, walking is easier, head and torso are carried erectly, and the foot movement is slimming to the ankles."[22]

Murray Pringle, in the pages of the May 1957 issue of *American Mercury,* also offered some fairly specific instructions in how to walk. So detailed were they that if one tried to follow them one would, of course, be thrown off stride and not be able to walk properly. Pringle advised using the heel-and-toe method: using correct posture, bending the arms at the elbow (just a little), and swinging the arms vigorously but naturally as one walked. To estimate speed, it was necessary for the walker to know the length of his stride, he declared. If the stride was 30 inches, 70 steps per minute would translate into about two miles per hour, while 106 steps equaled three miles per hour (said to be the pace maintained by soldiers), and 141 steps was about four miles an hour. However, Pringle urged his readers to aim for five miles an hour, around 180 steps a minute. Other advice included the need to buy shoes a half size too large, never to go for a strenuous walk immediately after a heavy meal, and wearing "white wool socks [that] are essential for walking any distance."[23]

Writing in the pages of the American Medical Association's official publication for the lay reader, *Today's Health*, Theodore Irwin argued in 1961 that the right way to walk was to be unhurried, unburdened, and prepared to stop and look at things whenever the urge arose. "Walk with your legs, not with the muscles of your back. Your toes should point straight ahead or even slant a little inward," he elaborated. "Relax when you walk. Let your legs swing normally and effortlessly. Permit your arms to swing naturally. Never hurry. Wear comfortable shoes."[24]

*Better Homes and Gardens* presented a breezy one-page article in its September 1977 issue that discussed "the four steps that can help you walk better and enjoy it more," or, in short, "how to walk happy." Point number one was for the walker to quicken his step with the advice to aim for 120 steps a minute, described as about four miles per hour while 130 steps was about 4.5 miles per hour. [Of course, that contradicted the earlier math from Pringle; however, this piece did not mention what length of stride it had in mind.] Point two was to lengthen the stride with the advice to note how many steps were taken to cover a measured distance and then to cover that distance in fewer steps. Third was the too obvious point to "wear proper shoes," with the readers advised not to wear platforms, sandals, or high heels when they set off on a walk. The fourth point was to "walk every day." The author of this article felt walking was a lot more enjoyable, and easier to engage in, if a purpose was involved, such as a walk to the library or to the supermarket. That is, the aimless, purposeless walk was not recommended.[25]

In a piece in *Glamour* in June 1978, reporter Jack Galub introduced, perhaps for the first time, the idea that walking was something one needed to prepare for prior to engaging in the activity; a warm-up was needed before a person could walk, just as a sprinter engaged in a warm-up before doing any sprints. Cited by Galub was William Gualtiere, an exercise physiologist, who advised people to walk three to five minutes at their normal pace to warm up and then to walk one to two minutes rapidly, slowing for one to two minutes, and so on. That slow-fast alternation was to be maintained for 23 to 25 minutes and to be done every other day. By the fifth or sixth week, thought Gualtiere, a person should be able to cover a half mile briskly (in seven to eight minutes) and in two months a full mile (13 to 15 minutes). After reaching that goal, the advice was not to strive for a faster pace but to extend the distance slowly, perhaps in one- to two-minute segments. At this point the warm-up concept was still in a somewhat rough and rudimentary form. It was around this time — 1978 — that walking fairly suddenly became faddish. A veritable blizzard of articles and books on walking appeared in 1979 and thereafter. And, of course, much of it concentrated on instructions on how to walk as the inherently simple and easy to understand was rendered complex and unfathomable.[26]

One of the first such articles appeared that year in the January issue of *Mademoiselle* with the lead advice being that walking 45 minutes a day could result in the loss of 30 to 35 pounds of weight in a year, although details were not provided. The idea was said to be for the reader to increase her usual two miles a day to five miles a day gradually over a period of several weeks, with the ideal speed being 12 to 15 minutes per mile.

Explaining away the math problem, the piece commented that everyone already walked two miles a day, roughly, around the office, and so on, so that going for a three-mile, 45-minute walk miraculously counted as five miles. A sidebar to the article recommended buying a pedometer (worn on the belt) because it "can change your life." And for its female readers who were not ready to wear their running shoes to work, the article showed three pairs of different "sensible" shoes that could be worn. As for the concept of contemplative solitude and the like mentioned by so many earlier writers on the topic, *Mademoiselle* argued, instead, "If you're walking to work ... find some friends to keep you company." Although this was among the first of numerous such articles, it incorporated many of the items that would become common to the genre: a preoccupation with gadgets, and numbers and a purely mechanical, instrumental view of walking that involved some questionable mathematics.[27]

A few months later, *Glamour* magazine profiled the activity of walking. Included in its dos and don'ts section were "Do have a destination," "Do break up a long walk with mental goals and landmarks along your route" [implying that walking was boring?], "Do wear comfortable shoes," and "Don't walk in a high-heeled pair." Then the article added its own complicated and unnecessary items by declaring, "Do tense your thighs and buttocks with each step for extra tightening benefits" and "Do move from the hips, not with your knees."[28]

*Mademoiselle* returned in July of that year with a longer article on the topic. After outlining the right way to walk, with a long list about posture, the piece declared the average walking pace to be two steps a second (120 per minute), or about three miles per hour with an average stride said to be 24 inches. [Most articles that spoke of a stride did not specify length but the few that had bothered had all used 30 inches as the standard.] How did one know if one's feet were properly positioned for walking, wondered the article? It answered by advising its readers to walk through sand, or with wet feet across the bathroom floor, then to draw a straight line between the footprints: "Ideally you should see a set of partial prints with toes that point just slightly outward ... and heels that come to within two or three inches of the line." Finally, the piece had a section on "Walking Warmup" complete with a series of exercises to do as a warm-up before one went walking. And the inane advice, the superfluous recommendation, had fully arrived.[29]

One month later, Abby Hoffman advised her readers that if they had any medical problems, or were simply over 40, they should consult a doctor before taking up walking. Like so many other advice writers of the time, she advised people to wear sensible shoes and not to walk in high-heeled shoes. Advising new walkers to work their way up to, preferably, 60 minutes per day, she was willing to accept two 20- to 30-minute periods as long as they produced at least 45 minutes per day. However, Hoffman counseled that anything less than walking at least three days a week and a minimum of 30 minutes a day would not yield much benefit. Hoffman, in keeping with a preoccupation with numbers and instrumentality, introduced a concept that soon became pervasive among walkers and those who supposedly instructed the masses through their books and articles. She advocated that the ideal exercising heart rate was 75 percent of a person's maximum heart rate. That maximum rate was 220 beats per minute minus the person's age. That is, the ideal exercising heart rate for a 50-year-old was 75 percent of 170 (220 minus 50), or 127.5. "Another aspect of a walking program that you should try to incorporate from the outset is a stretching and mobility exercise routine before and after each outing." The cool-down period had now been added to the warm-up. What had been a simple 30-minute walk in, say, 1970, had become a 45- to 50-minute chore in 1980. Then Hoffman listed three books on walking, two published in 1979 and one in 1978, observing, with no apparent irony, "All of the following books on walking contain a large quantity of self-evident material...."[30]

One of those 1979 efforts was *The Walking Book* by Gerald Donaldson. As it was one of the earliest books published on walking it was fairly light on self-evident material. It did not mention stretching exercises, either pre or post, nor did it urge the use of purpose-made "walking" shoes, although, of course, neither of those concepts had evolved at the time Donaldson would have been preparing his book. He did think that, while everybody walked differently, individual nationalities were thought to have certain characteristics; Italians walked with gusto, the French with style, the Germans with precision, the Dutch with deliberation, the Spanish with dignity, and the Scandinavians without inhibition. Donaldson's book was one of the few of a steadily increasing pile on the subject of walking that dealt with the past and the philosophy of the activity, at least to some extent. He cited Bertrand Russell as having once wrote, "Unhappy businessmen would increase their happiness more by walking six miles a day than any conceivable change of philosophy." Also, he cited a 1663 book — "*Youths Behaviour*"— in which the author Francis Hawkins laid down his commandments for proper walking. Included in that list were the following: "Move not to and fro in walking," "Hang not thy hands downwards," and "Kick not the earth with thy feet."[31]

An earlier 20th-century book concerned with instruction in the art of walking was the 1936 publication, *A Manual of Walking*, by Elon Jessup. He praised the activity because it was relatively injury free and people could continue walking into old age. However, his book was mostly concerned with long walks of 10 to 20 miles in the countryside and contained a substantial section on walking with burdens; that is, large packs.[32]

Milton Feher, who taught walking as the basis of dance at his school and had written a book on how to do it correctly, observed in 1980, "The two most common walking errors are tipping from side to side and tipping forward." Tipping forward, he added, was "probably the main cause of back problems in this country," while walking side to side instead of straight ahead "wastes energy and makes you tired."[33] A few weeks later, in the *New York Times*, journalist Jane Brody gave her advice on how to walk. She advised her readers to start slowly, to dress appropriately, to wear running shoes, to check with your doctor if you were just starting the activity, and "Don't forget to stretch" [that is, do a warm-up]. Perhaps the intellectual difference in the readers of the *Times*, compared to *Mademoiselle*, was the fact that in the former Brody apparently felt no need to counsel her readers not to wear high heels.[34]

*Glamour* magazine presented a three-month fitness plan in 1980 based on walking. A person started out in month one walking for five to 10 minutes three or four times the first week, and gradually built up the mileage. By the third week, the person was advised she should be doing three to four 20-minute workouts [walks] a week — with eight minutes of warm-up if a slow pace was used, 12 minutes of warm-up if a "training" pulse rate was used [that is, the by now ubiquitous heart rate at 75 percent of the maximum]. The goal at the end of month one was a 2.5 mile walk at a pace of 15 minutes per mile; goal at the end of month three was a five-mile walk at a 12 to 14 minute per mile pace. With no supporting evidence, the article declared a person walking would burn up as much as 80 percent of the calories a runner did and, "Walking provides better overall toning of leg muscles than you get from running." Such exaggerated statements as the last two reflected the over-romanticized and over-idealized image of walking that was sometimes presented when the activity was in fad status. It was, of course, something that often happened to anything that became a craze.[35]

*Current Health 2* advised in 1981 that stretching exercises be done before walking and a cool-down period undertaken afterwards. "The correct way to walk is to keep your head erect, abdomen flat, and back straight, while letting your arms swing loosely at your sides," went the counsel. "Move each leg forward along parallel lines, with the toes pointing straight ahead. Always land on your heel and roll to the outside of the foot."[36]

When *Consumers' Research Magazine* weighed in with a 1982 article, it advised the wearing of good shoes, of course, and, at that time, it still meant running shoes—walking shoes still awaiting invention by marketers. Down-to-earth with its advice, *Consumers'* did not mention stretching exercises, target heart rates, and so forth, but in indirect digs at others pointed out, with respect to walking, "Almost everyone can do it. You don't have to take lessons to learn how to walk" and "You can do it almost anywhere. All you have to do to find a place to walk is to step outside your door."[37]

Even a magazine as unlikely as *Mother Earth News* offered its own advice article on walking, in 1982. Included was a long section on what to wear, how to walk (for example, swing the arms rhythmically), and to use the 75 percent target heart rate. Also within the piece were discussions on the "talk test" and the "whistle test;" that is, a person out walking should be able to whistle while he ambled or to carry on a conversation with a companion. If a person could not perform either task he needed to slow down.[38]

*Mademoiselle* returned with a 1982 article that featured a six-week program for a person to build up speed and distance. This time around, tips for walking included "Don't walk after a heavy meal," "Try to keep your toes pointed in the same direction as your body," "Clock your distance with a pedometer," and "Take your pulse occasionally while you're walking." The latter point was made so the walker could see if his heart rate was at the appropriate target point. While the target heart rate was a straightforward concept, *Mademoiselle* managed to mess up the math. "To calculate your heart target zone first subtract your age from 200. This should be your maximum heart rate. If your pulse rate exceeds this number, you ought to slow down a bit, because you're pushing your body too hard," said the article. By subtracting a person's age from 180 the person was enabled to find the minimum heart rate with the advice that if the pulse was lower than that number, the person was not working hard enough and needed to speed up. Under *Mademoiselle's* interpretation of target heart rate, a 50-year-old's target zone was 130 to 150. That was a lot higher than the standard used by everyone else (220 minus 50 times .75 equals 127.5).[39]

Mary Ellen Pinkham, in the pages of *Ms* magazine in 1983, urged her readers to walk "before a meal or one hour after" at least five times a week. She favored using 70 percent of the maximum heart rate as the target zone. Additionally, she mentioned the "talk test" and the "sing test," in which the walker should "just barely" be able to sing out loud. Pinkham was also a believer in 10 minutes of warm-up time and 10 minutes of cool-down activity.[40]

By 1984, wrote reporter Bill Gale, the President's Council on Physical Fitness and Sports recommended that before walking "you should do about 20 minutes of stretching to ease your way into activity." Using the 220 minus age as the maximum heart rate, Gale suggested the walker elevate the heart beat to between 50 and 75 percent of that rate and keep it there for 15 to 20 minutes. In his opinion, 120 steps per minute equaled four miles per hour while 130 steps was about 4.5 miles per hour. Gale's unique contribution was to give complicated breathing instructions to his walkers: "Inhale as you take, say, four to six steps, and then exhale as you take your next four to six steps."[41]

In 1986, when Rosemary Ellis discussed fitness in *Working Woman* magazine, she observed that a well-constructed running shoe would work for most walkers but then hedged a little, in deference to new marketing concepts: "But other doctors recommend a shoe especially designed for walking." Ellis thought a warm-up was not necessary but a cool-down stretching period after walking was "definitely a good idea."[42]

Later that same year, *Mademoiselle* observed there were then aerobic shoes, running shoes, and walking shoes, "and all are different." Then it offered enough bizarre and complicated instructions in how to walk that would likely have turned many against the activity, including, "keep a body-conscious attitude, aware of your form and posture; breathe deeply, in through the nose and out the mouth, never huffing and puffing." Readers were also advised not to go out for a walk without (1) a visor, (2) a sweatband, (3) a sunscreen on all exposed areas, (4) lip balm with an SPF of 15, (5) a hair sunscreen. One was advised to take five to seven minutes each to perform warm-up and cool-down exercises (a list of four were provided). Instruction for the "stepout" [apparently the first step of the walk] was, "Leading with the right leg, reach out with the right hip, knee and heel to take a stride; your right heel should hit the ground first. Swing your left arm (bent at elbow) forward and your right arm back to propel you." Herein the target heart rate was described as "between 154 and 176 beats per minute minus your age," which should be maintained for at least 20 minutes. Once again, *Mademoiselle* had done poorly with the math. The result was not bad for a 20-year-old whose target rate by this method was 134 to 156. (Under the conventional standard, 75 percent, it was 150 and, 140-160 was 70 to 80 percent). However, it did not work well for the 70-year-old, at 84–106 (the conventional range was 105–120). For a 50-year-old, this math produced a range from 104–126 (only four years earlier a *Mademoiselle* article produced a range of 130–150), while the conventional 75 percent standard remained 127.5. What *Mademoiselle*'s odd math methods had in common was a seeming reluctance to force its readers to do a percentage; it appeared to prefer to present a single number, or range, from which an age could be subtracted, with no other math involved.[43]

Steven Jonas, a physician, started off his article praising walking as the most hassle free way to firm up muscles, lose weight, strengthen the heart, and keep blood pressure and cholesterol levels in check, and then declared, "Walk! Just put one foot in front of the other and you're off. There are no difficult techniques to learn, no expensive equipment to buy." However, his article then went on to be difficult, complex, and hard to follow, with the activity depicted as anything but simple. Jonas had what he called a new name for his technique of aerobic walking—"Pacewalking"—which happened to be the name of a book he had recently authored. According to him, the American College of Sports Medicine had determined that working out at 70 to 85 percent of the maximum heart rate for at least three times a week "will give you consistent health benefits." Jonas warned that a person could walk five miles a day too slowly and if the activity did not raise the heart rate into the target zone the exercise was of no aerobic use to the individual. Similarly, if one pacewalked—covering a mile in less than 12 minutes, for example, and putting the heart rate well into the target zone—and then simply stopped, there was no benefit. Even if a person walked a 12-minute mile four or five times a week, there would still be no aerobic benefit [that was because the exercise had to be undertaken for at least 20 minutes before stopping].[44]

Jonas then really began to complicate the "no difficult techniques to learn" concept. Since the idea of aerobic exercise was to efficiently use breathed-in air, he explained, "it's a good idea to learn how to breathe correctly." What followed were detailed instructions in breathing for the walker. Then a large spreadsheet was introduced, with the idea being for the walker to enter data, mostly number of minutes, in the cells. With respect to instructions on how to walk, Jonas declared, "Your fingers should be closed, not clenched" and "Your arms should be comfortably bent, at about a 90-degree angle. On the forward swing, your hand should reach a comfortable level above your waist. Then swing back and stop when you feel the muscles in the back part of your shoulder begin to stretch. For the first strike, come down first on the outside corner of your heel, then roll forward along the outside edge of your foot, pushing out with all your toes at the same time." More such instructions followed.[45]

Magazines aimed mainly at a male audience did not present many articles that included instructions on how to walk, compared to articles simply discussing walking as a craze. But the fad became so big that a few joined in. *Forbes* in 1988 started its piece by remarking, "Walking briskly and conscientiously is no status builder, but it can do a power of good." Noting it was not talking about race walking, "probably the only Olympic-class sport that provokes giggles" the article declared, "While you should swing your arms and legs to get maximum benefit, you don't have to learn a whole new way of walking. But you have to walk properly." *Forbes* advocated a target heart rate of 70 percent of the maximum. However, it added that it was not enough, even if one's heart was in the target, to walk 20 to 30 minutes at a time, three to five times a week, and expect a benefit. The average person, explained the story, needed to walk 4.1 miles per hour "in order to gain benefit from walking." But normal daily walking was reported to be done at only three miles per hour. It made the whole situation sound sort of hopeless. *Forbes* went on to say, "The only equipment you'll need are walking shoes that absorb the shock of walking better than running shoes can." Although it had promised its readers they would not have to learn a whole new way of walking, the piece then listed the book *Pacewalking* as a reference, which more or less did try and make the reader learn a new way of walking.[46]

Another male-oriented magazine, *Nation's Business*, briefly covered the topic, also in 1988. No mention was made of target rates, except to walk briskly (defined as a mile in 15 minutes). Stretching warm-up exercises were advised and, overall, this publication set very modest goals for its readership—"don't pick the closest parking stall for your car, pick one further away." Don't always use the elevator, use the stairs "at least one or two flights," and if one took a bus or subway then one was advised to get off one stop early and walk the rest of the way.[47]

*Ebony* magazine argued in 1990 that it was necessary to have a warm-up period, do stretching exercises [two separate pre-walking activities], and to have a cool-down period. "A brisk walk of about a mile a day is said to offer optimum cardiovascular benefit," which, of course, seriously contradicted some earlier advice.[48]

Marian Sandmaier touted the half-hour lunchtime walk for the working woman as worth the effort for that busy person. She said, "Walk naturally, with chin up and knees and hips relaxed. It's possible to burn more calories by bending each arm 90 degrees at the elbow and swinging them back and forth in a straight line (not across the body)."[49]

*Good Housekeeping* declared in 1992 that walking 30 minutes a day (not necessarily all at the same time) at a moderate pace of three miles per hour could burn an extra 120 to 150 calories a day, cause fat loss, and "Improve observational skills; total mental alertness (by improving overall circulation and oxygen levels in the brain)." It advised walking at a pace of three to 3.5 miles per hour and to achieve a target heart rate of 50 to 60 percent — using the lower percentage for a 60-year-old generated a pulse rate of 80, not much above a normal, resting pulse rate.[50]

Some of the silliest advice of all came in the pages of the trade publication *HR Focus* in 1993, for people who worked in the personnel area and did, among other duties, the hiring and firing of employees. It mentioned that Office Workouts, a Los Angeles-based provider of wellness programs for companies such as Xerox, Arco, and Pacific Bell, believed the single most important aspect of fitness walking was the stride, because maintaining a proper stride ensured a walking workout would be "safe and effective." To determine the proper walking stride, continued the article, "start by standing with your feet spread apart so that they are aligned with your shoulders. Slowly lean forward. Just as you're about to lose your balance, one foot will automatically move forward to stop you from falling. Let this happen. Then see how far your foot is from its original position. This is the length of stride you should keep throughout your walk." Once that was out of the way and the proper stride length determined, "take a practice walk around the neighborhood. You'll see a natural pattern of movement begin to develop with your arms and legs. As you walk, the right foot moves forward, then the left arm also moves forward, followed by the left foot and the right arm." After a mention of the talk test as a standard to keep in mind, the piece observed that breathing was important, with the personnel executive readership urged to "Inhale through your nose and exhale through your mouth."[51]

*Ebony* returned in 1995 to declare, "Experts say three 10-minute walking sessions a day are just as effective as 30 minutes walked all at once. You can park your car a few blocks from work and walk the rest of the way. You can walk during your coffee break, on your lunch hour, and to and from appointments." Such assertions were not then accepted by most authorities and represented an example of lowering the bar when the populace was perceived to be unwilling to meet the standard, but it was still the intention to deliver a positive and upbeat article. Readers of the piece were advised to start a walk with five minutes of stretching and to end with five minutes of stretching, presumably even for a walk during a coffee break. Complex instructions on how to walk included "Walk with your body in a natural upright position with your chin lifted and your shoulders held slightly back. With each step forward, plant your heel first, following through and pushing off with your toes. Try to keep your toes pointed forward rather than turning them inward or outward. Swing your arms gently at your side in opposition to your legs, bending them at 90-degree angles if you prefer. Your right arm and left leg should move forward, while your left arm and right leg move backward."[52]

Another somewhat unlikely publication with something to say on the topic was *Better Homes and Gardens*, in 1996. Reporter Kevin Knight mentioned the talk test, but in a different manner. If comfortable conversation was difficult, he thought, "then you're most likely conditioning your cardiovascular system." Knight felt you should not be able to chat continuously while walking and it was a good sign when you could not.[53]

It was not the case that the consensus on the talk test had shifted, for in 1997 in a general interest medical publication, reporter Tracy Early advised readers to take the talk test and if they found they were too out of breath to talk they needed to slow down. Early was one of many who advocated five minutes of stretching both before and after walking.[54]

Nowhere was the bar lowered more than in an article by Carol Krucoff that appeared in the *Saturday Evening Post* in 1998. She told the story of John Corrigan, who wanted to shape up but had no interest in changing his eating habits or joining a gym. Yet in six months he was able to drop 10 pounds and lower his cholesterol from 210 to 195, said Krucoff, "simply by taking a few extra steps at the office whenever he needed to use the restroom or get a bite to eat." Corrigan explained, "In the morning I'd walk to the cafeteria instead of using the machine near my desk." Added Krucoff, "Throughout his workday, whenever Corrigan wanted more coffee or snacks, or needed to use the restroom, he took the stairs to the basement instead of using the facilities nearby." Such a supposed success story caused the reporter to remark that we needed to restructure our thinking about walking and to keep in mind that every step counted. To that end, she offered tips that included: program your computer or alarm to remind you to take a brief walk periodically; a soccer mom could walk up and down the sidelines during her child's practices; and "Keep walking shoes in your car or desk so you can walk whenever you have a few extra minutes." Krucoff was as silent on why one would need special shoes for a three-minute walk as she was on the question of whether or not the person taking a three-minute walk should do five minutes of stretching before and five minutes of stretching afterwards.[55]

Suki Munsell, a "registered movement therapist" at the Dynamic Health and Fitness Institute in Corte Madera, California, said in 1999 that she did not like to encourage people to walk until they first learned to walk correctly. Where she worked, she taught "Dynamic Walking," "a posture-building walking method to help clients prevent pain." By this time technology had caught up with the heart rate target number and for around $100 one could buy a heart rate monitor that could be set so it beeped when the heart rate fell out of the target zone. Most brands contained a plastic transmitter and wristwatch display; an elastic strap held the transmitter over the heart area [perhaps just above the pedometer attached to the waistband, next to the water bottle?]. The transmitter detected the heartbeat and sent signals to the receiver wristwatch, which displayed the heart rate number and beeped, if necessary.[56]

Reporter Deborah King attended a "walking class" in London in 1999. Instructors became qualified to teach walking classes by attending a one-day Reebok workshop. King's class consisted of the group going for a five-mile walk in a nearby park.[57]

Christine Gorman praised walking in *Time* magazine in January 2002. As the new millennium arrived, walking continued to enjoy significant popularity and still had a certain amount of fad status, although it had diminished somewhat from the peak fad years of the 1980s and into the early 1990s. In her how-to-walk section, Gorman advocated walking shoes over running shoes and advised stretching exercises in both a warm-up and cool-down period. In a glib manner that made it far too easy for a non-walker to call himself a walker Gorman declared that some "shoehorn walking into their day by making minor adjustments in their daily routines, such as parking the car a few blocks away from the grocery store, taking the stairs instead of the escalator or prodding officemates to break for a walk rather than for a cup of coffee."[58]

All of the interest expressed in walking, which has waxed and waned over the years, had not led to much in the way of clubs organized by and for walkers (excepting mountaineering-type organizations). Nor had there been much in the way of official government promotion of the activity. Walk to work weeks have been rare, with conservation-minded governments more likely to promote carpooling, special high-occupancy traffic lanes, and better transit. Occurring more frequently have been direct and indirect references to walking and walkers as eccentric, as somewhat weird, as nerds, as losers, as lower class, and so on. The image of the walker has never been stellar or glowing, at least not in the 20th century. Unfortunately, sometimes the antipathy toward the walker degenerated into antagonism or hostility. And when it did it usually came from an automobile driver.

# 7

# Clubs, Governments, and Images

*"We believe that in the eyes of the law the pedestrian should always be right."*
                               Pedestrian League of America, 1959.

*"Walk a mile in the open air twice a day. It will add ten years to your life."*
                               New York City Health Department, 1906.

*"Walking is both a disgrace in the eyes of society, and a crime in the estimation of the officers of the law."*
                               Dr. Algernon Crapsey, 1912.

*"... people simply cannot believe that anyone is such a dunce as to walk by preference."*
                               Seymour Deming, 1916.

*"Walking is decidedly out of the mode; not only is it unfashionable, it is almost a sign of degradation...."*
                               Edmund Pearson, 1925.

*"A premeditating walker ... strikes most people as insane."*
                               New York Times, 1940.

*"Walking in the suburbs is social hara-kiri."*
                               Jeanne O'Neil, 1962.

*"Walking briskly and conscientiously is no status builder."*
                               Forbes, 1988.

An enthusiastic report in the *Los Angeles Times* in 1908 claimed that walking — the best and cheapest of all exercises — was undergoing an "astonishing" revival with men, women and children all over America said to be taking up the activity. "Walking clubs are being formed, business men are dismissing their carriages and auto mobiles and where the distance is not too great are going to their offices by way of the old-fashioned Shanks' Mare, and their employees are giving the laugh to crowded trolley cars and railway trains, with their fetid air and hoofing it," observed the journalist. Reportedly at Harvard, Yale, Cornell, and Princeton universities, walking clubs had been formed, as they had at other schools across the nation, with 10-mile jaunts by those groups being common. One inspiration for the increased interest in walking was said to be U.S. President Theodore Roosevelt. When he first came to Washington, said the account, "his love for walking was heralded from one end of the country to the other. His short, powerfully built figure became a well-known sight in the open country, just outside of Washington. A walk of ten miles was nothing for him...."[1]

Doctor John Finley was a well-known walker in New York City who had been involved in promoting walking as a government official in New York State's department of education and in 1925 was an associate editor of the *New York Times*. That year, he proposed people cover 1,000 miles in the open and on foot and that they join his fledgling League of Walkers to document their accomplishment and be recognized. To each of the first 1,000 people who completed the 1,000 miles by April 1, 1926 (some seven months in the future) and sent in a log—that is, an authentic record of the walks that totaled 1,000 miles, and included at least one single day's hike of at least 26 miles—Finley would send a bronze medal, the emblem of the League of Walkers. Finley remained a famous walker, having on occasion covered 60 and 70 miles in a day, and still walked around Manhattan Island once a year on his birthday. Apparently his proposed League of Walkers was short-lived.[2]

A British report in 1980 noted that the big increase in walkers in recent years had been among individuals and family groups rather than in organized parties, although the mainly rural Ramblers' Association had a 13 percent increase that year to a total of 35,700, while the more specialized Backpackers' Club, formed in 1972, had a membership of a little over 6,000.[3]

A 1998 report stated the American Volksport Association had more than 500 clubs nationwide that ran noncompetitive walking events outdoors. Still, interest in walking clubs seemed to be minimal. More commonly found, and covered by the media, were clubs of pedestrians formed to deal with the complex and antagonistic relationship that so often prevailed between walkers and automobiles.[4]

One such organization began to take shape in the UK in 1925 when a Dr. E. MacNamara was so appalled by the increasing "ignorance, stupidity, and reckless insolence" displayed by drivers toward walkers that he wrote to the *Times* (London) to state he would welcome and support something in the way of a pedestrians' defense league. That letter prompted a response just a few days later from N. Gasson to say that a Pedestrians' Protection Association (of which he was secretary) had recently been formed with the aims of maintaining and preserving the pedestrians' rights to use all streets, roads, highways, and so on, on foot and to use them in safety.[5] Apparently the Pedestrians' Protection Association had a short life and was gone by 1929. In that year an announcement in London, England, stated the Pedestrians' Association had just been formed to safeguard the interests of pedestrians. Lord Cecil of Chelwood was president of this new group, and this one would last.[6]

Formal organization of the Pedestrians' Association did not occur until November 1929, when it held its first meeting and drafted a memorandum to the UK Minister of Transport. At that meeting, Lord Cecil explained he got the idea for the group in the spring and summer of 1928 when he attended a parliamentary inquiry investigating the automobile industry but found no one there to represent the interests of pedestrians. In the Pedestrians' Association memorandum to the transport minister the first thing they asked for was "that some test should be imposed on drivers before they were allowed to drive." Of special concern to them were the number of deaths and injuries to pedestrians from traffic accidents. In describing those accidents at their inaugural meeting, the group used such phrases as "a calamitous holocaust of pedestrian life" and "wholesale destruction of pedestrians."[7]

In a dismissive and sarcastic editorial in the *Times* (London) Lord Cecil was patronizingly called a "romantic idealist" and, while the editor criticized the behavior of both drivers and walkers, he reserved most of the vitriol for pedestrians. In conclusion, the editor declared the best thing the new organization could do would be to train its members and the general public in the duty of looking where they were going.[8] In 1938, the Pedestrians' Association issued a leaflet entitled "Pedestrian Crossings: Advice to those who use them." The leaflet was part of a nationwide campaign for securing the better observance of pedestrian crossings; a campaign said to be endorsed and commended by the UK Minister of Transport.[9] When it commented on the Greater London Council discussion paper, "Traffic and the Environment," in 1972, the Pedestrians' Association asked the Council to appoint a pedestrian commissioner to give advice on pedestrian movement and requirements. Positive planning was needed, argued the group, to make walking easier and pleasanter in London by means of walkways, and traffic-free streets. Also requested were improved bus services and a ban on trucks in local streets.[10]

A group of mainly elderly pedestrians who bounced cars off pavements in protest at the "car culture" won the backing of a UK government minister in 1995. Steven Norris, the junior transport minister, said that several anti-car groups were living in "fantasy land," but, he said, the Pedestrians' Association, which had joined with several new groups in taking action against cars, traffic levels, and exhaust fumes were "within their rights" to push cars off sidewalks. Members of the group descended on a street in Tufnell Park in north London and pushed cars from sidewalks into the road. Norris, though, admonished a group called Reclaim the Streets, which a month earlier had blocked off a north London high street with scrap cars. "The Pedestrians' Association is not simply the elderly chapter of Reclaim the Streets," explained Norris. "What they are doing is very sensibly pointing out that many short journeys do not have to be made by car." Pedestrians' Association chair Faith Lawson (in 1973 the group reportedly had 1,000 members but more recent numbers were not available) was delighted with the support. "We have been campaigning for donkey's years to improve the walking environment and make it safe," she said. "We have won a few points but not changed government policy radically. It still deals with the symptoms not the cause, which is too many cars."[11]

Still in existence in 2001, the 72-year-old Pedestrians' Association decided its name was a little dull, perhaps, and therefore renamed itself Living Streets. Organization director Ben Plowden said, "The word pedestrian is, it seems, a serious turn-off. People are unhappy because of its negative associations." Plowden explained he wanted to see the group reach out to the younger generation and abolish its image of "being a group of car-phobic fogies waving walking sticks at pavement cyclists." He admitted the group (with 1,500 members) had declined since its 1930s heyday, when he claimed it was instrumental in forcing the introduction of the driving test, compulsory car insurance, and the 30 mile per hour urban speed limit.[12] Back in that heyday period of the 1930s, an account in *American City* remarked that organizations of pedestrians for the main purpose of reducing the hazard to which walkers were subject were becoming "increasingly powerful" in England and on the European continent "and bid fair to rival the great motoring clubs in the near future." Two of the best known were said to be the Pedestrians' Association and the Verkehrswachten (Traffic Vigilantes) of Germany.[13]

Many years later, in 1959, the Pedestrian League of America was founded by Joan Vickies, a former Philadelphia safety official, and Leo Wilensky, then director of the League. A year later, the New York City-based organization said it had 150 members in 10 states. Declaring his group was not anti-automobile, Wilensky added, "We are out to insure the pedestrian's right to walk. The first Pedestrian League was organized by members of the Woman's Christian Temperance Union during WWI, but it directed most of its efforts against drunken driving. This is a far cry from what we are trying to do" now, he said, "which is to watch out for the safety, health, freedom, and economic welfare of pedestrians." Part of the group's philosophy was, "We believe that in the eyes of the law the pedestrian should always be right. We consider the jaywalking laws unconstitutional. The pedestrian should be king of the road." Wilensky argued further that the automobile prevented the pedestrian from exercising his freedom of movement and the air pollution caused by automobiles infringed on his freedom to breathe properly. Noted by a reporter was the fact that none of the League's administrators owned or drove cars, which made them, he thought, "peripatetic saints."[14]

Almost two years later, the same reporter made a return visit to the Pedestrian League of America and Leo Wilensky. Unhappily he observed, "The American Automobile Association has seven and a half million members; we have about a hundred and eighty" and "We get anonymous harassing letters, saying, 'Don't go too far in your advocacy of....'" He lamented there was no one else; "there are thousands of pro-motorist groups but only one group that speaks for the pedestrian." Wilensky was also annoyed by one of the dictionary definitions of the word pedestrian—the one defining it as commonplace. "There is a great need for improvement in the dictionary field. 'Pedestrian' is not even listed in some encyclopedias," he complained. Said the reporter, "Mr. Wilensky was alternately optimistic and depressed, generous and severe, and our spirits rose and fell with his." Disappointed in the lack of growth in membership, Wilensky concluded that "the results are disappointing. We accept no donations—to avoid corruption. And no salaries. We used to forbid our officers to have cars; now ownership of cars is restricted to forty per cent of the officers. We want to avoid any conflict of interest; we don't want members who are in the auto industry or belong to automobile clubs."[15]

Fourteen months after that the reporter returned to interview Wilensky for the third time, who thought the pedestrian was as much of an underdog as ever. Recalling the League's "early" days in 1960, he said the group was on the radio, on television, in movies, in magazines, and in newspapers, all at once. "We received letters, invitations to speak in Philadelphia," he continued. "Then there was a blackout. Everything stopped. I just can't forget it. The automobile industry, it's a billion-dollar industry. The fact that most of the daily press censors and distorts the news in the industry's favor shows how powerful it is." No more was heard of this group.[16]

A 1963 announcement stated an International Federation of Pedestrians had been formed in Brussels to study issues around the "education and protection of pedestrians" and to secure common action on matters of common interest. Delegations from Britain, France, Holland, and Belgium attended the foundation meeting, with T. C. Foley, secretary of the British Pedestrians' Association elected secretary of the new organization.[17]

Very little information with regard to official government (at any level) promotion of purely pedestrian interest was ever reported, probably because very little of it ever took place. Back in December 1906, the New York City Health Department announced it was attempting to organize the city into I.W.W. (I Walk to Work) groups. Prospective members were admonished to "walk a mile in the open air twice a day. It will add ten years to your life. If you don't believe it try it and see." Climax of the week-long campaign was an eight-mile walk on Sunday, December 10 — the "Finley Hike" — with the state's commissioner of education, Dr. John H. Finley, promising to award medals and prizes to winners of the Finley Hike, cosponsored by the city Department of Health.[18]

In its editorial on I.W.W. week, the *New York Times* declared, "To whatever degree they succeed in this attempt, to the same degree will they raise the general average of urban health, for there is no doubt that New Yorkers ride more, and walk less, than they should." That was thought to be because New Yorkers lived a great distance from work, had several means of public conveyance to get them there cheaply, quickly, and comfortably, and "the usually unresisted impulse is to take a car. This results not only in lack of needed exercise, but in the breathing of bad air through the greater part of the day." Reportedly, over 200 people participated in the campaign ending Finley Hike, "many of them women." Groups represented in the hike included members from the Walkers' Club of America, the Ladies Walking Club of America, the American Walkers' Association, and the women's division of that organization.[19]

Several years later, in 1921, Finley, chairman of the League of Walkers, (but no longer New York State Commissioner of Education) returned from a trip to Europe filled with a desire to start an active campaign to popularize walking. On the ocean liner going to Europe, Finley said he walked upwards of 100 miles on the ship. He lamented the fact that the U.S. was so far behind Europe in its appreciation of walking.[20]

During the 1960s in Canada, the federal government resolved to do something about what it saw as the sorry state of the average Canadian's level of fitness. A popular idea of the time was that the average 60-year-old Scandinavian was in better physical shape than the average 30-year-old Canadian. To remedy the situation, the Canadian government introduced a program called Participaction — that included a walking component. Medical giants like Dr. Wilder Penfield put their weight solidly behind a "walk for pleasure and health" program then under way across Canada. A new national Council for Walking was formed by the government, with its first publication, a booklet entitled "Walk for Pleasure," available to the public for free.[21]

July 1, 1973, was declared by the U.S. government to be Walk a Mile for Your Health Day, with U.S. Senators William Proxmire and Mike Mansfield walking around the Capitol grounds in Washington, D.C., to urge Americans to participate. President Richard Nixon put his personal stamp of approval on the observation of Walk a Mile for Your Health Day, with the event sponsored and promoted by the President's Council on Physical Fitness. Nixon's remarks on the event included the following: "I know from personal experience that long walks are refreshing exercises of the mind as well as the body. It offers time for reflection and time for personal thought."[22]

Antagonistic attitudes toward walkers and walking can be found from earliest times. Dr. Algernon Crapsey of Rochester, New York, did some long-distance walking — up to 20 miles a day — in 1912. He reported that "walking is both a disgrace in the eyes of society, and a crime in the estimation of the officers of the law." Apparently he had a run-in with the police, but he provided no details. Crapsey declared, "The man who walks is considered an idiot or a pauper. If he has not the money to ride he is a vagabond, and if he has the money to ride and does not do it he is looked upon as a fool. That one would walk for the mere pleasure of walking seems no longer comprehensible to the average man or woman." On his jaunts, Crapsey walked from one small town to another.[23]

A reporter by the name of Seymour Deming commented in *Atlantic Monthly* in 1916, "In railway and streetcar belts people simply cannot believe that any one is such a dunce as to walk by preference."[24] Two years later, in 1918, an article in a Canadian magazine celebrated gasless Sundays — then recently introduced in Canada as part of the war effort to save gasoline — because the writer loved walking. However, he did admit, "To profess a love for walking is now almost as singular as to profess a belief in astrology or the political sagacity of William Jennings Bryan."[25]

An editorial in the *Times* of London in 1923 assessed the class differences involved in walking and how that helped shape attitudes toward the activity. Noted was that walking on a big scale was once part of a poor man's necessity and he walked, not as in 1923 for the pleasure of walking, but because it was his only means of getting from place to place. Few rich men walked more than short distances and "going for a walk" was a phrase little used in that earlier time. As transportation got cheaper and more accessible, that attitude changed as walking became a deliberate occupation of the leisure hours. So swift and widespread was that change, thought the editor, that the "great walks"—often within living memory—which were part of the normal routine of peasant life "appear now as chapters of a remote legend."[26]

When journalist Edmund Pearson discussed walking in 1925, he thought one reason a city man was afraid to walk was the worry he would be taken for a rube. If he were seen taking the stairs he feared he might be thought ignorant of "the blessings of science; it may appear that he does not know about elevators, or that he distrusts them; that he is, in short, guilty of the great American sin of not being up to date." Pearson added, "Walking ... is decidedly out of the mode; not only is it unfashionable, it is almost a sign of degradation ... and the American waist-line is steadily growing in circumference."[27]

As mentioned earlier, open hostility to walkers was obvious in the 1929 editorial in the *Times* of London in response to the efforts of Lord Cecil to form the Pedestrians' Association — the sole organization to lobby for walkers' concerns in the face of many such groups devoted to motorists. "The pedestrian very often is wrong, and it is the more stupid of him because very often he owns a motor-car himself," it said. "But the stupider he is, the more necessary it is to protect him against his own stupidity" and that of people like Lord Cecil, who "attempt to divide mankind into two irreconcilable classes, of which one is all guilt and the other all innocence."[28]

So bizarre was walking considered by some that there were examples where authorities had imposed it as a punishment. A compulsory long walk was imposed in Afghanistan in 1933 on some Afghans who spoke unfavorably about conditions in the south of the country. They were sentenced to go and see for themselves, walking about 1,000 miles, with escorts and placards describing their offense and punishment. Discussing the unusual sentence, a British newspaper editor commented, "Also, like much else that is penitential in character, walking is good for the health, and the prisoner at the end of such a sentence is likely to be a stronger as well as a better informed Afghan."[29] In response to the Afghan story, a man by the name of F. Haynes of London wrote to say that in his early days at Eton he was sent on a walk to copy the inscription on Queen Anne's statue at the foot of Windsor Castle as a disciplinary measure, and later was sent all the way up the "Long Walk" to copy the inscription on George III's statue. Haynes did not know if the practice still continued at Eton.[30]

Edward Foster, 16, pled guilty in 1935 to participation in the robbery of a grocery store at Alexandria, Indiana. Judge Charles E. Smith, at the courthouse in Anderson, Indiana, gave the boy a choice of a term in a reformatory or a "walking" sentence. Foster chose the latter, which called for him to walk a round-trip every day between Anderson and Alexandria (12 miles one way) for 60 days, except Saturdays and Sundays when he only had to hike one way. Specific conditions required the trips to be made solely on foot with no hitchhiking allowed. On his first trip it took him three hours and 45 minutes to cover the 12 miles. Also, on each walk he had to carry a 20-pound load, which represented the weight of the goods stolen from the grocery store. Smith's strange sentence was brought to the attention of Governor Paul McNutt at Indianapolis, but he said he saw no reason to interfere, arguing the youth had accepted the walking punishment over a term in a reformatory. Grace Swords of the Anderson Humane Society had discussed with representatives of the Anderson Council of Women the possibility of launching a protest against the conditions imposed on Foster, but no formal action was taken.[31]

When a *New York Times* editor tackled the subject in 1940, he began by declaring, "The whole history of mankind suggests that the human animal, as such, does not like to walk. His idea of progress ... has been to avoid walking. He has ridden every kind of animal that would stand to be hitched." Then he went on to assert, "A premeditating walker, who not only does not thumb for a ride but will not accept one, when offered, strikes most people as insane. People who walk usually feel obliged to offer an explanation: they are looking at birds ... or else they need the exercise. Few of us dare to say that we walk because we like to walk." One suggestion offered by the editor was that there could be more provision for safe places to walk, especially along country thoroughfares, where speeds were high "and many motorists regard the pedestrian as a blot on the landscape."[32]

Reporter J. M. Flagler observed in 1958 that nobody walked in America and the few who did came under scrutiny; "Indeed, there are sidewalkless communities where the police look with suspicion upon anybody who isn't riding, and many a suburban prowl car has pulled up and cruised significantly alongside the Stories [a couple fairly well known at the time who systematically walked the city streets of various cities]."[33] According to writer Peter Steinhart, at different times writers Aldous Huxley and Ray Bradbury were stopped and questioned by Los Angeles police because they were out walking at night. Bradbury recalled his interrogation later in a story. The police could find no good reason for a writer to be out walking at night even after he explained he was "walking for air. Walking to see." They replied, "You have a viewing screen in your house to see with," and took him away. Bradford Ketchum of *The Walking Magazine* commented,

"Walking is not macho. You can't get teenagers to do it. And people look at it as boring."[34]

Writing about the suburban situation in 1962, Jeanne O'Neill remarked, "Walking in the suburbs is social hara-kiri. If you want to be snickered at by the neighbors and snubbed by the PTA, just go out and take a walk. Or try to. Actually, you won't get very far. Somebody you know, or somebody you don't, will drive up and insist upon giving you a ride. Nobody believes you're walking because you want to. In Suburbia, dire necessity is the only thinkable mother of ambulation." Perhaps in order to emphasize that she was not an oddball, O'Neill carefully explained she did not have a "thing" about walking: "In most respects, I'm a normal, sedentary, noneccentric, unremarkable suburbanite. It's just that, every once in a while, I feel like taking a walk. And it makes me mad as Ophelia that I can't." She added, "If ordinary walking is inviting the head shrinker, walking in the rain is psychotic.... But I'm fond of my children and I don't want them to miss out on parties, so I drive to the other side of town for rain-walking."[35]

After journalist Robert Thomas Allen lamented the drive-in culture in a 1963 piece, along with a sit-down culture that featured items such as golf carts and rider mowers, he said, "We used to take our girls for a walk. Any girl today who had a boy call on her and ask, 'Do you want to go for a walk?' would figure she had gotten stuck with a failure."[36]

Joseph Wood Krutch brought up the issue of class in 1964 when he mentioned that Thorstein Veblen attributed the loss of interest in walking to the supposed fact that members of the leisure class refused to use their legs in order to demonstrate that they did not have to—as in China where the deformed feet of female aristocrats were status symbols proudly displayed to show that if they wanted to go anywhere there would always be someone to carry them. In George Bernard Shaw's *Pygmalion*, the newly created lady who had just been asked by an admirer if he could walk her home through the park demonstrated her sense of newly acquired status by explaining, in words more appropriate to her former lowly station in life, "Not bloody likely. I am going in a taxi."[37]

Reporter Deidre Carmody interviewed people in 1982 who walked to work in New York City. Impetus for the piece was the release of 1980 U.S. census data on the percentage of people who walked to work. Although Carmody's article was presented straight, the underlying tone was that these people were quaint, at the very least. She spoke to several people who used the Brooklyn Bridge as a pedestrian route to Manhattan. What seemed to fascinate her was the clothing sworn by female walkers. "Here she comes: the ultimate, sophisticated New York career woman. Her hair is coiffed, her makeup impeccable. She is wearing a silk blouse, a dark blazer, a slim, expensively tailored skirt — and thick, white woolen socks and rubber-soled running shoes." Carmody added that "there was a time when an elegantly dressed woman wearing running shoes would have been associated more with Bellevue [a psychiatric institute] than with Bloomingdale's but along came the 1980 transit strike and changed all that."[38]

High-status magazine *Forbes* acknowledged in 1988 that walking could do a person a lot of good, but added, "Walking briskly and conscientiously is no status builder."[39] In 1993, journalist Taki Theodoracopulos wrote about the joys of walking, which he discovered when he had to give up jogging for a few months following a knee operation. At the age of 55 he recalled the poor image of walkers: "When I was a schoolboy, walkers were considered the [Bill and Hillary] Clintons of the time. They were the wimpy ones who did not go out for sports, excelling instead in theatrical pursuits, and whose girls during the prom weekend resembled young Barbra Streisands."[40]

Jane Holtz Kay was the author of the book *Asphalt Nation* (about the evils of car dependency). While promoting that book, she was challenged about the fact she was a car owner herself. So she sold her car, rendering her family a car-less household. Then she wrote a lengthy 1997 article about her adjustment to that status. The very fact she would write such an article and get it published was in its own way a testament to the status of walkers in America. "But whatever the wearisome aspects of walking and mass transit, of being viewed by skeptical friends as an eccentric Mary Poppins wafted by air, I had an easy answer to any predicament in my car-free life," she wrote, meaning the $6,000 she was saving each year by not owning a car. Kay's article had the tone of somebody doing something eccentric and how others might follow her lead since it was not hard to do, but very much in the quirky or oddball category. She reported that in the previous five years "my car-free lifestyle has begun to look less oddball." Reportedly, only nine percent of American households (mostly poor) did not own a car.[41]

When author Bill Bryson returned to live in America in 2000 after 20 years in the UK, he settled in the small town of Hanover, New Hampshire, and got around a lot on foot, by choice. "People have gotten used to my eccentric behavior, but in the early days acquaintances would often pull up to the curb and ask if I wanted a ride," he reported. Bryson added, "We will go through the most extraordinary contortions to save ourselves from walking. Sometimes it's almost ludicrous." As an example, he cited a woman who complained to him about the difficulty in finding a parking spot in front of a local gym. She went there several times a week to walk on a treadmill. At most, the gym was a six-minute walk from her front door. When he asked her why she did not walk to the gym and do six minutes less on the treadmill, she replied, "But I have a program for the treadmill. It records my distance and speed and calorie burn rate, and I can adjust it for degree of difficulty."[42]

But there were benefits to be had from walking according to many sources. Some of the benefits were true, some were exaggerated, and some were false. Broadly speaking, those benefits could be divided into two general categories: mental (psychological and mood) and physical (health and medical).

# 8

# Benefits of Walking — Mental and Psychological

"I'd recommend a 10-mile walk as a good post-election antidote."
Dr. W. H. Thompson, 1940.

"Walking is an exercise in intellectual development."
Dr. Harry J. Johnson, 1962.

'[Walking is] a way to get fit, save the planet, make our cities livable, have a little fun — and it's all for free."
John P. Wiley Jr., 1989.

At the beginning of the 20th century, journalist Arnold Haultain wrote a long, glowing piece in *Atlantic Monthly* on walking in which he declared that a walk, especially a country walk, was a "mental tonic." When a person went off on such an excursion, concluded Haultain, "You get away from rivalries and trivialities; from scandal, gossip, and paltriness ... you get away from barter and commerce, from manners and customs, from forms and ceremonies; from the thousand and one complications that arise when a multitude of hearts that do not beat as one try to live in a too close continuity."[1]

During the time of World War I, Andrew Fenn, who walked 10 miles a day, listed the physical benefits from walking that would come to be more or less standard: it sharpened the appetite, aided digestion, contributed to sound sleep, aided blood circulation, and toned the entire system. Mentally, he asserted, walking cleared the mind, drove out worry and increased one's general efficiency, while esthetically the activity opened up a new world as it revealed nature at first hand. "The main regret of one who walks is the scarcity of fellow enthusiasts," lamented Fenn, "and the inability to confer the pleasures and benefits of walking ready-made upon one's doubting friends." Around the same time Seymour Deming argued that one who walked, "instead of seeing more than he can take in, takes in more than he can see." For him, "wisdom is gathered on foot, along country roads." While ideas could be gathered anywhere, they should be tested "on the road."[2]

Writing in 1936, James Kerr called the first three decades of the 1900s "the speed age," but was reassured by what he saw as the revival of the "ancient art" of walking. Not just walking instead of taking transit but walking "for the sheer joy and love of it." Kerr was especially enthusiastic about country walking, where Nature became a person's teacher "and from her you will learn who you are, and what is your special quest in life, and whither you should go. You relax in the presence of the great healer and teacher, you turn your back on civilization, and most of what you have learned in schools and colleges."[3]

Fulsome in her praise for the activity was journalist Juliet Pickett, who declared in 1938, "Walking has more powers than I dare claim for it, lest I seem like the barker at a medicine show and attest so much for this elixir that my customers will turn away!" Besides the healthful benefits of walking Pickett enthused over its broadening aspect from exploring nature and the brain clearing of introspection on a solitary sojourn, or the social benefits of companionship if not walking alone. The ledger on walking, she summarized, showed not a single red entry. "Yes, walking is clean, healthy fun. It entails the smallest monetary outlay per hour of happiness that can be found," she concluded. "It is the password to a green world of peace and measured beauty."[4]

Another who liked the escape value of walking was Donald Peattie, who observed in 1942 that while a person was out walking he could not be reached by telephone or telegraph and the walker could not reach anyone in those ways. He saw that as a great blessing and added, "You cannot put out a hand, as you do even in an automobile, and twiddle the radio.... You cannot play bridge or consult an astrologer, bet on a horse or go to a movie." As compensation for those "keen deprivations," Peattie argued that walking offered "health, happiness and an escape from civilization's many madnesses."[5]

In the wake of Franklin Roosevelt's re-election as U.S. president in 1940, Dr. W. H. Thompson, head of the philosophy and psychology department at the University of Omaha said, "I'd recommend a ten-mile walk as a good post-election antidote" for those worried about the election. According to Thompson, the frontal lobes of the brain became overactive when the fear mechanisms were aroused, and mild exercise, such as walking to the point of real fatigue, tended to lessen the severity of the images, the fears called up.[6]

A golden rule in the eyes of an editorial in the *Times* of London in 1955 was "After supper walk a mile." It was an activity that was said to hold calm delights, although the editor admitted the temptations to ignore the rule were many, and it was likely not observed by that many people. Waxing eloquent about the man who did follow this golden rule the editor asserted, "He takes his walk easily with a fine sense of release from the pressure of the day ... and a man may choose without compelling distractions to think about anything or nothing."[7]

Supposed mental benefits from walking began to get more specific — and more exaggerated — in more recent times. Carlos Fuller in 1959 reminisced about the time he was a young man who taught school in a rural schoolhouse. He walked each way, six miles a day, about 1,000 during the school year. On those walks, he began to concentrate on ideas for school, studied poems, thought about books he had read, wrote things down in a notebook he carried, and so on. "Through it all I learned to drive away dull hours by establishing the habit of harnessing my thoughts to life-giving ideas," he declared. Through the following years, Fuller added, he used in public speeches and written papers material that he grew to understand or had memorized on those country walks.[8]

Dr. Harry J. Johnson, president of the Life Extension Foundation went so far as to say in 1962, "Walking is an exercise in intellectual development. When you are out walking, you have no choice but to think." That caused reporter Jeanne O'Neill to lament that walking was out of fashion and perhaps too healthy, like spinach, to be popular. "Anything that keeps your muscles in tone, aids your respiration, digestion and circulation must perforce be unpleasant," she stated. "Or maybe it's too easy, and readily available." During a Manhattan bus strike the previous spring, many people were forced to get out and walk. One former bus rider told O'Neill that walking was healthier, cheaper and took exactly the same amount of time as did the trip by transit, but, he added, "You know, I'd keep it up even after the strike — if only it weren't so much trouble."[9]

Robert Rodale, of Rodale Press and *Prevention* magazine, wrote in 1988 about a type of walking that the century did not have time for, a type of walking that many great thinkers and dreamers of the past would not have missed. He called it "strolling," while others referred to it as "sauntering." In any case, it was slow walking meant for meditation and observation and renewal. It consisted of a lot of aimless rambling and pausing — along a moonlit beach, for example; "it stretches the spirit instead of the sinews." Like other types of walking, strolling regenerated the person, not by helping the person lose weight, or by lowering the blood pressure as more vigorous walking might, "But by clearing your head for creative thought." Thus Rodale advised his readers to take a stroll regularly, but not as a replacement for faster-paced walking, rather as an essential part of a personal walking program. Secondly, he advised people to get twice as much out of their strolling by creating a "stroll guide"—that is, a journal.[10]

Joe Gibson wrote in 1991 that he had never had a driver's license. When he was asked by people how he managed without a car, he pronounced himself puzzled by their puzzlement. His article was as much an anti-car piece as it was pro-walking, with Gibson arguing there was an essential passivity about driving that found its cultural equivalent in television, which also claimed to provide access to a larger world. "In fact, neither activity demands more than a constant partial alertness and a narrowed focus; both require passivity and stasis." On the other hand, said Gibson, "Walking deepens perception, allowing the mind to construct and organize experience into a meaningful pattern as it happens." He urged his readers to "Try it sometime — unplug the television, leave the car keys on the table and step into the dance of nature. You will not regret it. Indeed, you may end up walking everywhere."[11]

Writing in *Architectural Record* in 1992, Stephen Kliment delivered an editorial in praise of walking in which he commented that walking, for the architect and the student, was more than a means of transportation; combined with observation, walking was a teacher of many things—planning, urban design, materials, details, textures, colors under different lights, sociology, and zoning at work. For Kliment, perhaps the greatest virtue of walking was that, for the most part, buildings and neighborhoods were still designed to be seen at the walking pace of 3.5 miles per hour. It was impossible, he thought, to take things in by any other means, such as on a bicycle or in a car: "Trying to take in the urban scene by car is even less rational [than being on a bike]; it's like eating a shrimp with a pitchfork: the scale and dynamics are lacking."[12]

Mark Bricklin, in an editorial in *Prevention* magazine in 1996, stated there was a lot of evidence that regular exercise like walking could do wonders for a person's head, yet only a small number of therapists seriously encouraged their patients to partake of this "natural medication." That was a message he said he got after talking with psychologists who had done research in that area, or who used "walking therapy" as part of their practice. According to Bricklin, those people argued that regular walks provided the following benefits for a person's head: helped lift depression, lessened tension, reduced confusion, increased optimism and hope, boosted self-esteem, and increased energy. To get those benefits, those experts were said to generally recommend walking almost daily, for 30 to 60 minutes each time.[13]

Jay Walljasper, in 2003, wrote an old-style article about the joys of walking that was a throwback to articles of 100 years earlier. This editor of the *Utne Reader* asked rhetorically why he was going to do more walking with so many crucial matters in the world crying for attention. He implied that some of the world's problems could lie with politicians, military generals, company CEOs, and the like, who spent all their time in offices and automobiles and never in walking. Walljasper then cited the 18th century social critic Jean-Jacques Rousseau, agreeing with the latter's comment — "When I stop [walking], I cease to think; my mind only works with my legs."[14]

Walking was even said to make managers more productive and efficient and, of course, to ultimately produce more profit for their employers. For a time, walking programs designed especially for managers were quite the vogue. One program for managers, administrators, and so forth, called a "walking rally," took place in Billund, Denmark in 1980. Participants' employing companies had paid substantial fees in the hope that, faced with the uncertainties of 10-kilometer night walks through unfamiliar territory, their managers would "learn to observe reality, distinguish fact from fantasy and begin to work together as a team." The basis of the program was team training and team thinking propounded by Jiro Kawakita in his book *Teamwork*. The method was modified — and provided with its walking component — by Shigeru Kobayashi, who ran walking rallies in Japan under the auspices of the Japan Management Center. According to reporter Roy Hill, Kobayashi devised the walking rally "as a means of getting people to experience practical difficulties, see those difficulties factually without opinions intruding, then to think, plan and reach consensus before taking any decisions." Participants in the rallies were divided into groups of eight to 12 people, who were then paired up within the groups. Each pair embarked on a night walk, using maps that were basically accurate but that gave somewhat sketchy information and could be misinterpreted. Also involved were timed checkpoints and point losses for mistakes.[15]

The U. S. trade publication *Supervision* (for managers, foremen, and supervisors) presented an enthusiastic article on the benefits of fitness walking for its readers in 1988. According to the piece, walking could release tension, provide an outlet for pent-up emotions and release hormones and blood fats that were harmful if they remained in the body. Reporter Sallie Stephenson concluded by informing the supervisors that "A good walk can bring you back with your energy supply renewed and your haunting anxieties will be dispensed. It can be more useful than the tranquilizers and pep pills that Americans swallow by the billions each year."[16]

Link Up, a UK industrial recruitment agency with 150 permanent staff in 23 offices and 2,000 temporaries on its rolls, decided in 1995 that its monthly staff meetings were boring, stifling, and needed to reinvigorate themselves. So Larry Gould, chairman of Link Up, decided the next senior management meeting would be held on a 12-mile walk. Simon Ward, a fitness instructor, was hired to organize the first executive hike for 10 managers, seven of whom were women. Gould pronounced the first walk a success and declared the walks would be a regular event, although the next walk was limited to seven miles as 12 was determined to be too far. Also, said Gould, "stopping off for croissants and coffee only two hours into a six-hour walk was too soon."[17]

Such group programs were even sometimes extended to cover all employees. Bethlehem Steel (Pennsylvania) had a noon-hour walking program for its employees in the early 1990s, and by 1992, 550 of the 5,000 employees at Bethlehem's home office and plant participated in the program. After each program's 10- to 12-week duration, participants were given evaluation forms. Results from the 30 percent of walkers who returned the questionnaires indicated that 52 percent of the participants lost weight (from one to 20 pounds); 19 percent lowered their blood pressure; 16 percent lowered their cholesterol level; 63 percent felt better about themselves; 40 percent felt better able to handle stress; 24 percent influenced the other employees to exercise; 19 percent improved their eating habits; and 99 percent expressed interest in participating in another walking program.[18]

Rosemary Ellis told the readers of Working Woman in 1986 that since she had started to walk to work, "the first 40 minutes of the day are mine. The phone doesn't ring, my thoughts flow uninterrupted."[19] According to exercise physiologist Joan Gondola and psychologists at Baruch College in New York City, "as fitness levels increased there were positive personality and mood changes." Added Gondola, "We do know that the better your fitness levels, the greater the self-image and self-esteem. With women especially, we've found that as their fitness levels improve, they become more extroverted and have more friends."[20]

Patricia Bleyle stressed the benefits of mental well-being in Ms in 1988, from what she called the "walking cure." She said that although walking was then making a strong comeback as exercise, to be considered therapy, "it cannot take place just anywhere and in any manner. The swish, swish of cars and buses on city streets, the dense distractions of materialism at the mall, and the tinny sounds of a Walkman radio will distract you from walking's psychotherapeutic value." Her definition of walking therapy was as follows: "the sustained and regular rhythm of solitary movement through the countryside." Generally, she argued, any form of psychotherapy was expected to increase the sense of well-being, efficacy, and self-respect. It should also give a better perception of reality, shore up courage, and awaken the senses. "I claim that for many people walking will contribute to all of the above," declared Bleyle. It was also true, she wrote, that for walking to be of use as a therapy, it had to take place in the woods and the fields—not anywhere near civilization—"where the walker can celebrate the present moment in the sound of the cock's crow."[21]

More fanciful than most were the claims made in 1989 by reporter Lilly Dickson, who declared—but offered no evidence—that walkers reported improved eyesight, healthier gums, a rosier complexion, and enhanced self-esteem when they were on a regular walking program.[22]

That same year, a completely different benefit from walking was cited by John P. Wiley, Jr. First, though, he quoted a line spoken by a noblewoman in Emily Eden's 1830 novel *The Semi-Attached Couple*: "It would kill any of the young men of the present day to attempt such a walk; it must be four miles, or two, or some immense distance." Claiming that was a relevant sentiment 160 years later when he was writing, he extolled walking by saying, "Here's a way to get fit, save the planet, make our cities liveable, have a little fun—and it's all for free." Walking was a way to exercise, he stressed, that did not require adding a whole new unpleasant chapter to each day; something that could be done without special equipment or going to a special place, "Something that lessens the damage being done to the planet we love." Wiley argued for city walking to the extent of perhaps five miles a day but he was quick to point out that those miles did not have to be all done at once. Concluded Wiley, "We can do something about global warming, and feel better for doing it. Each time one of us walks someplace instead of driving, that much less poison has been injected into the air we all breathe."[23]

When *Ebony* magazine discussed walking, in 1990, it quoted Dr. Deborah Bernal, chair of the National Medical Association's physical medicine and rehabilitation section and professor of medicine at Howard University Medical School, as having said, "Walking has definitely increased in popularity. I know I've been advising it. It's catching on among Blacks, particularly women." One of the reasons for its new popularity, thought *Ebony*, was that it was "a safe exercise." According to this publication there were five major benefits from walking: weight loss, improved cardiovascular health, strengthened bones, stress reduction, and improved attitude and mental functioning.[24]

Writing in *Current Health 2* in 1997, journalist Tracy Early listed a myriad of benefits said to be obtained from walking; it prevented the possibility of getting diabetes because people in your family had it, lowered cholesterol levels, reduced the appetite, was practically an injury-free activity, increased the length of life, improved heart health, toned and strengthened muscles, reduced stress levels, promoted weight loss and kept it off, helped to avoid high blood pressure, improved blood flow and circulation.[25]

California State University at Long Beach psychology professor Robert Thayer had spent much of his research time on the study of moods, culminating in his book, *The Origin of Everyday Moods*, in 1997. For people who were tense, tired, depressed and edgy, the best way to improve the mood was to raise the energy level—"go take a walk" was his recommendation. For him, the obvious mood enhancers such as caffeine, cigarettes, food, alcohol, and shopping provided only a short-term solution because they left you feeling worse later on. According to his research, even socializing, listening to music, or reading a book were only moderately uplifting. A 10-minute brisk walk, on the other hand, could boost energy and act as a kind of tranquilizer at the same time, he claimed. In Thayer's view, maximizing energy and minimizing tension was the goal, and exercise accomplished that. Reporter Gail Vines remarked, "For today's sedentary citizens, the beauty of Thayer's ideas is that even a little exercise can do you good. You don't need to be physically fit to reap the psychological payoff." Frank Eves, who lectured in applied psychology at the University of Birmingham in the UK observed, "More exercise isn't better, psychologically-speaking ... little bursts of 10 minutes are certainly a much more realistic option for sedentary people" than 30 minutes all at once.[26]

While a considerable number of people touted the mental and psychological benefits derived from walking, there were more who hyped the health and medical benefits.

# 9

# Benefits of Walking — Health and Medical

*"[For every hour spent walking] you can tack on another hour to your life, and perhaps one or two more hours as well."*
                                    Stanford University researchers, 1986.

*"It's simple, it's cheap, and studies show that walking may be the best exercise for reducing the risk of heart disease, stroke and diabetes.... Walking, in fact, may be the perfect exercise."*
                                    Christine Gorman, 2002.

In 1923, American physician Alvah H. Doty, a former health officer of the Port of New York, admonished his fellow Americans to walk for health, indeed for life. He maintained that the tenure of life depended upon the soundness of the blood vessels, especially those of the brain. "It would be difficult," he wrote, "to conceive of a simpler and more effective protection against undue internal blood pressure than walking," both for its simplicity and its efficacy. Doty believed the value of walking was minimized by the public, "for it is a human failing not to appreciate aid which we may obtain without effort or expense." To derive any benefit from the activity, remarked Doty, it had to be indulged in daily and systematically. Golf, tennis, and so on, were not equivalent to a daily walk, he continued, because there was more to walking than physical exercise, "Walking stimulates the mind, especially walking in congenial company."[1]

That same year, another U.S. medical doctor (unnamed) wondered about the people who were so lazy they drove everywhere instead of walking, and asked if America was "going to become a physically lazy nation, and, through lack of exercise, a people of pendulous abdomens and small legs?" Calling walking one of the best forms of exercise and one of the best ways of keeping healthy, he noted that it often prevented obesity and cured many cases of indigestion. "A walk a day, from three to ten miles, should be a health rule for everyone," he urged. Women, he argued, often consulted a physician because they were fat and wanted to lose weight; they dieted and followed every fad, "yet they are leading exponents of a sedentary life. They hate to walk. When they are advised to walk to reduce their weight they invariably say that they can not because their feet are sore." The doctor attributed that to wearing fashionable shoes that ruined the feet.[2]

Dr. Frank J. Monaghan, health commissioner of New York City, released a statement in which he discussed exercise during the summer season of 1925. One piece of advice he offered was, "A form of exercise which everybody can enjoy daily is walking."[3] At an annual meeting of osteopaths held in London, England, in 1925, Dr. Hubert Pocock (from Toronto) told the assembly that not only was walking on tiptoe an effective remedy for some ailments, but also a preventive. Diabetes, he added, was one of the diseases walking on tiptoe would help. "Watch the gorilla and you can see how the human frame can best be supported," concluded Pocock. "The gorilla's tremendous chest is the result of its posture. Men must learn to walk on their toes."[4]

Not everyone endorsed walking as an effective weight-reducing tool. Mrs. Thomas Havercamp decided the activity was not a good way to lose weight and she resigned in 1935 as one of the few female letter carriers in the U.S., having walked about 34,000 miles since 1920 in the service of the U.S. Postal Service. "And," she explained, "I weigh forty-five pounds more than when I started."[5]

Dr. Paul Dudley White, who went on to become a renowned doctor, argued in 1937 that the current "fads" for hiking and bicycling should be transformed into permanent features of America's daily life, not only for the sake of health but also for enjoyment and economy. He regarded regular daily exercise in moderation as a valuable health measure, "even though one can survive without it and still live to an old age." According to White, adequate muscular exercise relieved mental fatigue, cured insomnia, and helped prevent constipation; further, heart disease and high blood pressure were less common in those who maintained a habit of daily exercise and avoided obesity than in those who took no exercise. It was the soft physical life of the adults of modern times that seemed to be undermining the health of many hearts in America, he declared. For economy's sake it was cheaper and more efficient for people to walk, cycle, or take transit to work, thus lessening congestion and traffic problems. White advised that walking or cycling a few miles a day should suffice for health benefits and "should be regarded in the same light as eating and sleeping, as an essential part of the day's program." While he wanted to see more people walk two miles or cycle five (in 30 or 40 minutes), he felt a change was needed to permit the cyclist and pedestrian to travel in safety, such as the addition of dedicated cycle paths like these that then existed in parts of Europe.[6]

Dr. Paul Dudley White, a heart specialist and vice president of the American Heart Association in 1940, seemed to be in favor of more vigorous exercise when he urged Americans to turn from "excessive" use of automobiles to "walking and cycling" so the automotive industry could devote itself more fully to national defense work. Such a change would also be a boon to the health of Americans, said White, because he was convinced from his own medical practice that one of the great errors of the day was the failure to take regular exercise. During the past generation, emphasized White, "the American people have developed a habit of excessive use of motor cars ... and individuals have utilized them almost as a part of their body, giving up the simpler means of locomotion such as walking and cycling."[7]

Writing in *Hygeia* (an official publication of the American Medical Association directed at the lay reader) in 1944, journalist George Weinstein argued that at age 35 or 40, people should give up all active sports that involved sudden starts, stops, changes in direction, stiff competition, and so on, as they were all too hard on the heart. "So stow away your tennis sneakers, your handball gloves, or your gym membership card; instead, climb into a good, stout pair of walking shoes," he urged. With respect to stories one might have heard that contradicted his advice, such as that of the king of Sweden who still played tennis at age 85, he said to forget them: "Just remember that the United States Army, which has studied the problem thoroughly, does not want men over 37." However, said Weinstein, "Walking is no sissy exercise," and could provide almost as stiff a workout as a set of tennis. For men and women aged 35 to 40 and over, walking, he declared, rated as "the perfect exercise" that was an excellent foot and leg conditioner; it also strengthened stomach muscles, took inches off the waistline, toned up the muscles of the upper body and improved posture. In conclusion Weinstein observed, "Walking can also be a good cosmetic. There is no better 'skin food' than speeded-up circulation which brings to the inner layers of the skin nutritive elements."[8]

A study of American youth by Dr. Hans Kraus, associate professor of medicine at New York University, in 1956, was brought to the attention of President Dwight Eisenhower. Results disclosed that in six tests given to groups of European and American children for physical fitness, 57.9 percent of American youngsters failed one or more of the tests as against only 8.7 percent of the Europeans. Investigators believed the difference lay in the fact the European children were more physically active. Instead of being taken to school by bus, for example, they walked.[9]

Journalist Murray Pringle observed in 1957, "Medical authorities advise sedentary workers to walk five miles a day in order to reach a ripe old age. Most car-owning Americans don't walk five blocks in a day!" Veteran walkers, he maintained, seldom suffered from fatty heart, jumpy nerves, or double chins, and regular brisk walks also stimulated blood circulation, a good preventive of leg and foot trouble.[10]

Dr. Harry J. Johnson, medical director of Life Extension Foundation (a firm that, among other things, conducted annual health exams for some 20,000 executives of some 500 companies), advised moderation in all things. Johnson walked from home to his office — a distance of two miles — but only if it was not raining and the temperature was above 20 degrees Fahrenheit, which he cited as an example of his definition of moderation.[11]

After a much publicized heart attack around 1964, actor Peter Sellers told reporters his doctor advised him in the future to walk three miles every day and to take a nap each day after lunch.[12] William Fitzgibbon told the subscribers of *Reader's Digest* in 1972 of the benefits of walking. He commented that Abraham Lincoln had been a great walker and that Thomas Jefferson called walking "the best of all exercises," even though the precise physical benefits of walking were then unknown. But modern medicine had discovered them, "and today doctors make assertions about the benefits of brisk walking that have a sound basis in medical fact." Fitzgibbon emphasized, "It is not mere walking that they are talking about — it is brisk walking," although he did not define the concept. It was around this time, roughly, that the instrumental view of walking began to come to the fore and eventually to dominate; that is, only a certain type of walking had any value (fast, more or less) and from there came the development of applying mathematical equations to the activity of walking, such as the heart target zone number. While these increasingly "scientific" concepts were applied to walking, the amount of time people were required to walk (as advised by experts) was continuously lowered to match the seeming needs of a populace too lazy to do very much of anything. Striding, as Fitzgibbon termed his brisk walking, improved blood circulation, cleared the mind, improved the disposition, and cut fatigue. "Experts are cautious about making claims that daily striding will increase one's life-span," he said. "There is no hard proof that it will, and the most that experts will say is that with brisk daily walking you can remain youthful in condition, if not in chronological years." Also cited was Dr. Paul Dudley White, who said "A vigorous five-mile walk will do more good for an unhappy but otherwise healthy adult than all the medicine and psychology in the world." From this time onward it would become increasingly rare for an authority to advise his readers, in a mass circulation magazine, to go for such a long walk. In the 1990s, for example, it was unusual for an expert to advise people to take a five-mile walk on a regular basis.[13]

An advice article in *Changing Times* in 1972 declared that medical opinion held that adults needed exercise equivalent to about four miles a day on foot. Bizarrely, the author of the piece then stated, "Letter carriers, housewives and others who are on their feet most of the day already walk more than this, and even office workers normally cover a mile and a half."[14]

Jack Galub started his 1978 article by commenting, "Medically recognized as a means of coping with low-grade depression, walking can lift your spirits. When properly done, it also triggers weight loss and helps enhance your cardiovascular fitness level, especially when you learn to include stairs and hills." Galub then went on to introduce the 70 to 75 percent target zone number. According to him, the maximum heart rate was 200 beats per minute at 20 years of age, decreasing one beat per year (for example, 190 beats per minute at age 30, 160 at 60 years of age). The idea was that exercise should push your pulse, or heart beat rate, to 70–75 percent of the maximum (140–150 beats per minute in a 20-year-old), and that exercising to bring the heart rate to, or near, the maximum was both unnecessary and impossible. [No evidence was presented that the maximum heart rate decreased in the stated fashion, or that the number 200 was accurate in the first place, nor that 75 percent was the ideal target, as compared to, say, 90 percent or 60 percent]. Cardiologist and internist Dr. Borisse Paulin agreed that raising the heart rate was important to cardiovascular fitness enhancement: "If the heart is made to beat within this zone for a half-hour or more a day, its stamina increases. In fact, the total cardiovascular system becomes more efficient." Paulin added, "A brisk half-hour walk can help you lose weight because you feel better and, as a result, you tend to eat less."[15]

*Changing Times* ran another advice article on walking in 1980. Cited were the usual health benefits from the activity and the plan of the President's Council on Physical Fitness and Sports was to put more status into walking. As an example of decreasing standards, the presidential council then recommended a goal of walking three miles in 45 minutes and a minimum of three such walks per week.[16]

Charles Kuntzleman argued in 1980 that a brisk half hour of walking helped a person lose body fat (which he said differed from weight), that medical authorities declared exercise could be more relaxing than medicine, and "walking reduces the chances of your getting a heart attack." While Kuntzleman brought up the concept of target heart zone, the numbers he used were to elevate the pulse to 70 to 85 percent of the maximum rate. Also, he was one of the first to introduce the concept of the "talk test" mentioned earlier, that is, as a person walked he should be able to hold a conversation with a person beside him. If he could not then he was walking too fast for his age and fitness level.[17]

According to reporter Joan Lippert in 1981, if you walked briskly enough and for at least half an hour at a time, walking became an aerobic exercise like running, swimming, cycling, ice or roller skating, disco dancing, and cross-country skiing. "This means it can improve your circulation, benefit your heart's pumping ability and your lungs' efficiency, and fortify the network of blood vessels throughout your body just as well as more strenuous aerobic exercises," she added. Dr. Kenneth Cooper (then the guru of aerobics, and a book author) said brisk walking could give your body the same training effect benefits as any of the more strenuous exercises, it just took longer. To meet Cooper's weekly goal a person had to walk 2.5 miles in 33 minutes five times a week, as compared to running two miles in 18 minutes four times weekly, or biking six miles in 21.5 minutes four times a week, or swimming 800 yards in 15.5 minutes four times weekly. Robert B. Sleight, executive director of the Walking Association in Arlington, Virginia, said, "What other sport allows so much togetherness and so little competitiveness? People who walk together talk together.... You don't have to worry about injuries." Nathan Pritikin, the man behind the controversial Pritikin program for diet and exercise said he believed that daily walking, coupled with his diet plan, could reverse heart disease.[18]

According to Dr. James Rippe in 1986, cardiologist and director of the Exercise Physiology Laboratory at the University of Massachusetts Medical School, "For the past thirty to forty years orthopaedic surgeons, cardiologists—even the Army—have performed studies on walking that have shown us it has real long-term health benefits." That caused journalist Kristin Donnan to tout the activity as an easy, effective alternative to swimming, cycling, and so on. And that it could provide a person with most of the benefits of a more strenuous sport like running with virtually none of the risks. Among those benefits were increased muscle tone, weight loss, and improved cardiovascular and respiratory fitness. In yet another example of lowered standards, Donnan declared a person could reap all the benefits available from the activity by walking for 20 to 30 minutes, three to five days a week. No mention was even made by Donnan that the walking should be at least brisk. At the low end of her numbers, a person had to walk only a total of 60 minutes in a week to receive all the benefits— about four miles in total.[19]

Some 12,000 men who were at risk for developing heart disease participated in a health study during the 1980s. During seven years of follow-up, researchers at the University of Minnesota School of Public Health found that those men who were moderately active in their leisure time had 30 percent fewer deaths from heart attacks than more sedentary men. In particular, the decreased chance of dying was associated with light- and moderate-intensity activities: that is, walking, as well as cycling, bowling, fishing, gardening, yard work, home repairs, dancing, and swimming, for example. According to the researchers, the duration of activity necessary to make a difference was only 30 to 69 minutes a day. Studies showed a regular walking program lowered blood pressure and the resting heart rate. University of Minnesota researchers also said exercise might lead to a longer life by helping people maintain their proper body weight. Reporter Susan Zarrow added, "A brisk walk steps up blood flow to the brain, making clearer and more creative thinking, some studies suggest."[20]

Researchers at Stanford University, also in the 1980s analyzed the lifelong exercise habits of a large group of men. For every hour spent walking, they concluded, "you can tack on another hour to your life, and perhaps one or two more hours as well." Said Robert Hyde, one of the study's researchers, "We found that men who walked nine or more miles a week had a risk of death 21 percent lower than those who walked less than three miles a week." Men who walked 30 to 35 miles a week seemed to get the optimal amount of exercise, with their death rates cut in half. Investigators also found that when men walked more than 35 miles a week, death rates began to slowly rise again. Such results caused reporter Gale Maleskey to use the following for an article subhead: "What miracle treatment can help alleviate heart disease, diabetes, obesity and depression? It's as simple as putting one foot in front of the other." Maleskey enthused that researchers had found that brisk walking could lower blood pressure, help people lose weight without dieting, improve blood fat levels, reduce the need for insulin in people with adult-onset diabetes, relieve back pain and headaches, and even improve mood and thinking skills. Endocrinologist Dr. Robert Levin told his patients (mostly older women with osteoporosis) that walking would improve their stamina, stability, muscle tone, and bone density: "It will improve their quality of life."[21]

David Levitsky, a Cornell University professor of nutritional sciences said, "A single life time walking habit could probably prevent much of the weight gain people see as they get older." Other researchers at the University of Minnesota found that HDL (high-density lipoproteins), blood fats thought to help protect against heart disease, rose significantly in obese young men who walked briskly for 90 minutes, five days a week, for 16 weeks. Said Dr. Arthur Leon, main researcher on the study, "If you also lost weight while you were exercising, the effects on HDL levels were twice as good." Men in that study lost about 25 percent of body fat with the walking program. Their insulin requirement also dropped by 43 percent. At the Hypertension Clinic at the University of Florida in Gainesville, daily walking was recommended for everyone. Dr. J. Robert Cade, professor of medicine there, commented, "Brisk walking definitely controls blood pressure better than drugs for some people."[22]

Researchers Larry Tucker and Glenn Friedman measured the association between walking for exercise and the ratio of total cholesterol/HDL cholesterol in 3,621 adults in 1990. After controlling subjects for age, gender, income, body fat, alcohol use, exercise other than walking, and cigarette smoking, adults in the high (4.5 hours or more of weekly walking for exercise), moderate (2.5 to 4.0 hours), and low (0.5 to 2.0 hours of weekly walking for exercise) duration walking categories were compared to those in the no walking, no exercise category. Findings revealed that adults who walked for exercise 2.5 to 4.0 hours or more each week had less than one-half the prevalence of elevated total cholesterol/HDL rates than those who took no exercise or were in the low duration walking category. Concluded the researchers, "desirable total/HDL ratios may, in fact, result from moderate to high levels of exercise walking ... at least 2 1/2–4 hours of exercise walking per week should be practiced for protection against elevated total/HDL ratios. In this study, 1/2–2 hours was not associated with decreased risks of high total HDL ratios."[23]

According to Dr. Steven Blair of the Dallas-based Institute for Aerobics Research, people who were out of shape did not need to attain an athlete's level of fitness to avoid a high risk of death. People could pull themselves out of the high-risk group, he said, by simply going for a brisk walk for 30 minutes to an hour, five days a week. Athletes exercised at 90 percent of their maximum heart rate to achieve the level of fitness they needed, while joggers worked at 80 percent of capacity, explained Blair: "People who exercise for health, however need only work at 40 to 60 percent." Said Blair, "When you walk, you control weight, lower blood pressure, and reduce cholesterol and blood sugar. Walking also helps reduce stress and may improve the quality of your sleep.... For people over age 60, there is an even stronger relationship between the level of fitness and reduced cardiovascular disease and cancer."[24]

A new study in 1991 claimed to show that regular hour-long strolls (that did little to improve cardiovascular fitness) could nevertheless reduce a woman's heart disease risk by boosting her blood levels of high-density lipoproteins (HDLs), which helped remove cholesterol from the body. It was said to be the first clinical study to show that exercise need not be vigorous to lower a person's risk of cardiovascular disease. Researchers took 59 healthy, sedentary premenopausal women and divided them into four groups: aerobic walkers who exercised at 86 percent of their maximum heart rate; brisk walkers, 67 percent; strollers, 56 percent; and a sedentary control group. The three walking groups covered 4.8 kilometers (three miles) a day, five days a week, for 24 weeks. From before and after measurements, investigators concluded that while fitness increased in direct relation to walking pace, HDL levels rose the same six percent whether the women strolled leisurely or "power walked." That HDL increase should slash a woman's cardiovascular disease risk by 18 percent, study leader John J. Duncan of the Dallas-based Cooper Institute for Aerobics Research, estimated.[25]

Cardiologist James Rippe, director of the exercise physiology lab at the University of Massachusetts Medical School, prescribed a simple two-step plan for people who wanted to feel better and reduce their risk of heart disease: "Eat cereal with skim milk for breakfast, then go out for a 15-minute walk." He added, "Exercise doesn't have to be something tough and sweaty and separate that you do. Like brushing your teeth or taking a shower, exercise can fit into your daily routine as a general maintenance for your body."[26]

A pilot study conducted by the College of Nursing at the University of Oklahoma Health Sciences Center targeted full-time female employees in a large Oklahoma City company who were overweight and sedentary. A control group was established along with an experimental group that attended eight weekly support group meetings, received weekly walking assignments, and completed weekly walking diaries. Study leader Deborah Booton explained that "we chose this activity because it has been shown to have a positive impact on many actual and potential problems. It is also a very manageable activity, even for overweight and sedentary women." After eight weeks the women in the experimental group had lost a significant amount of inches from their waist, hips, and thighs. However, no significant changes were found in the weight, blood pressure, cholesterol, and body fat percentage between the two groups. A follow-up one month later found those subjects who had continued walking reported a greater satisfaction with themselves, their jobs, and life in general, while members of the control group did not have increased satisfaction in any area.[27]

Evan Thompson reported in 1994, to a presumed upscale readership in *Canadian Banker*, that a major 1992 study found that even a brisk half-hour walk daily protected most people from cardiovascular diseases and cancers as well as a range of other maladies that circulated throughout the workplace. However, Thompson said the average person took 25 minutes to walk one mile and that a 20-minute mile was considered to be "brisk." Both were off the mark; 15 minutes or less was brisk while a 20-minute mile was a stroll.[28]

In a year-long study in 1995 of 238 healthy postmenopausal women (average age 62) those who habitually walked an average of just a mile a day had seven percent higher bone density in their legs and four percent higher bone density overall than women who walked less than a mile a day. According to epidemiologist Elizabeth Krall, who conducted the study at Boston's Human Nutrition Research Center at Tufts University, there was no difference in bone density between women who walked 3.5 miles twice a week and those who walked seven miles in one outing. "It doesn't matter how you break up the walking, as long as you do it at a fairly brisk pace — about 15 minutes a mile."[29]

When a major study released its results in 1998 after 12 years of research, it found that covering just two miles a day cut the risk of death almost in half for people in their 60s, 70s, and 80s. Amy A. Hakim and others from the University of Virginia calculated that every mile older people walked daily lowered their death rate by 19 percent. Despite such oft-reported results, most Americans did not engage in walking or any other exercise. Dr. Jody Wilkinson, medical director of the Cooper Institute for Aerobics Research, said 60 percent of Americans did not get enough regular activity to improve their health, with the numbers thought to be worse for the elderly. The research for this study was based on the Honolulu Heart Program, which had followed the health of 8,006 men of Japanese ancestry, 61 to 81 years of age and living on Oahu since 1965. Of those who walked more than two miles a day, 24 percent died over the 12 years of the study, compared with 41 percent of those who walked less than one mile daily. The walkers' risk of death from cancer was especially lower, as those who walked infrequently were about 2.5 times more likely to die of cancer than were the men who walked at least two miles a day.[30]

A large study that looked at the benefits of walking in reducing heart disease among women issued results in 1999 that stated exercise did not need to be strenuous to produce significant results. Three hours of brisk walking per week, or half that time spent at jogging, aerobic dance, or other vigorous exercise reduced the risk of heart disease 35 to 40 percent, the study of 72,488 women aged 40 to 65 over eight years reportedly found.

But the walking had to be brisk (defined here as three miles per hour) to be effective, strolling did not work, no matter how long you walked. Walking briskly for five hours a week was said to cut the risk of heart attacks by 50 percent and even 1.0 to 2.9 hours of brisk walking brought a 30 percent reduction in heart attacks and deaths from other coronary problems.[31] From that study it was also determined that the 20 percent of the women who exercised the most were only 54 percent as likely to develop adult-onset (type 2) diabetes, as were the 20 percent that exercised the least. Among women whose only activity was walking, the 20 percent who walked longest and fastest were only 58 percent as likely to develop diabetes as the 20 percent that walked the least.[32]

Another 1999 study looked at 2,678 men aged 71 to 93 and found those who walked 1.5 miles a day had half the risk of heart attack compared to those who walked only 0.25 mile. Still another study of 6,000 men aged 35 to 60 found those who walked 11 to 20 minutes a day were 12 percent less likely to develop high blood pressure than non-walkers, but men who walked 21 minutes or more reduced their risk by 30 percent.[33]

Journalist Christine Gorman produced an article for *Time* magazine in 2002 that was full of praise for walking. "It's simple, it's cheap, and studies show that walking may be the best exercise for reducing the risk of heart disease, stroke and diabetes." According to Gorman, walking should be done for a half hour or so at a time, maybe five or six times a week and at a "reasonably vigorous clip," which she defined as three to four miles per hour. "Walking, in fact, may be the perfect exercise," she enthused. Dr. JoAnn Manson, chief of preventive medicine at Harvard's Brigham and Women's Hospital, remarked, "If everyone in the U.S. were to walk briskly 30 minutes a day, we could cut the incidence of many chronic diseases 30% to 40%." Yet, said Gorman, less than one-third of the adults in America got the recommended amount of exercise each day, and 40 percent were almost completely sedentary. Gorman's article then went on to list some of the areas in which scientists were said to have already identified health and medical benefits to be derived from walking. It was a long list: (1) heart disease — as much as a 50 percent reduction in the risks of suffering a heart attack; (2) stroke, reduction in risk; (3) weight control; (4) weight loss; (5) diabetes — brisk walking could postpone or prevent its onset; (6) osteoporosis prevention; (7) arthritis — walking reduced the pain by strengthening the muscles around the joint; (8) depression, easing of; (9) cancer, perhaps a lowered risk for some types but Gorman admitted the evidence there was weak and further study was needed.[34]

All those scientific studies that purportedly showed a multitude of benefits from walking began to appear in the late 1980s, about a decade after walking caught on as a fashion with the public as a form of exercise. That fad, which quickly became a craze, started around 1979. It was partly driven by medical reports trickling out that walking was medically beneficial, and at the same time drove researchers to produce more studies. Walking had formally arrived as an exercise, rather than an activity everyone had always engaged in, albeit in widely varying amounts of time and distance. Once so redefined, it needed, of course, a coterie of experts to interpret, explain, and make pronouncements.

# 10
# Walking Reborn as a Trendy Exercise

> *"You might be tempted to say 'Walking is not really exercise, it's ... well, it's just walking.'"*
> Current Health 2, 1981.

> *"No one has discovered a fountain of youth, but a lifetime walking program will certainly slow the physiologic aging process."*
> Robert Sweetgall, 1985.

> *"The mall walkers are attracted by a large space heated in the winter and cooled in the summer, where there is no traffic, where the surface is smooth and conducive to walking and where there are no fears about safety."*
> William Stockton, 1988.

One of the few early commentators who insisted walking was an exercise and not just an activity, with its own set of rules, was New York Health Commissioner Dr. Royal S. Copeland, who said in 1922 that a fat person need not expect to lose weight until he or she moved so briskly that perspiration was induced. And not artificially-induced perspiration, but what he called "honest sweat." He declared that, while walking was a splendid exercise, one had to walk briskly and long enough to produce the desired amount of perspiration. "Sauntering on the shady side of the street, stopping to look in the shop windows, or sitting down now and then on a park bench, will do absolutely nothing towards removing fat," he explained. "Even if you should walk five miles in this manner every day, you wouldn't lose weight." To the contrary, he argued, that type of "gentle" exercise acted as a stimulant to the appetite and, consequently, could result in increased weight.[1]

However, such walking, or any type of pedestrian activity, lacked followers or popularity for much of the 20th century as the automobile dominated American life and dictated locomotion styles. Lynn Waldorf, University of California football coach, and Eddie Wojecki, head trainer at Rice University in Houston (he had been head trainer of the 1952 U.S. Olympic team), observed in 1955 that just a few years previously, early football practices were exercises aimed at loosening knee muscles, but it was just the opposite in 1955, with exercises designed to tighten the muscles. The two men ascribed the change to "the great decrease in walking, occasioned by the habitual use of cars and the simultaneous decline of hiking."[2]

When Bernard Rudofsky wrote *Streets for People: a Primer for Americans* in 1969, he decried the lack of walking in the U.S. To an American, he said, walking was the "most undesirable" way of locomotion: "The very idea of walking — beyond the necessity of getting to and from his car, or of covering the distance from a subway station to his office — is distasteful to him." In Los Angeles, Rudofsky continued, a man walking on the street without a dog equalled a bum, and "Policemen may not be able to recognize a bank robber when they see one but are not fooled by the stride of a dedicated walker, and many a man who went for an airing ended up at a police station. In California, walking is regarded as an antisocial activity." According to a Los Angeles Planning Report he cited, the pedestrian "remains the largest single obstacle to free traffic movement." At that time, in Portland, Oregon, it was unlawful for any person to "be upon the street, alley or public place" between the hours of 1:00 and 5:00 a.m. without having and disclosing a lawful purpose. When that ordinance was challenged, the court was unable to conceive of a situation where a "sane" person could be upon the street without "some purpose."[3]

Well-known Olympic runner Abby Hoffman authored an article on walking for *Chatelaine* magazine in 1979. It was a piece solicited by the publication and was an effort to cash in on a fad then just taking hold. After mentioning the many books that had been published on the subject in the previous year or two, and the fact that walking had become a craze, Hoffman stated, "Undoubtedly some of the claims [for its benefits] are wildly exaggerated, but the fact is that we are finally coming to accept a cheap, enjoyable and eminently practical way to better health and better feelings about ourselves as physical beings." Hoffman argued that serious fitness buffs had been quick to heap scorn on walking as a form of exercise because they said it was not sufficiently challenging physically, but that was wrong.[4]

Writing in the unlikely forum of *House & Garden* in 1981 (indicating the spread of the fad), journalist Suzanne Murphy said that, according to

U.S. government estimates, more than 45 percent of the U.S. population was physically inactive. Such people ran higher risks for various health problems and the federal government wished to remedy that. Said C. Carson Conrad, executive director of the President's Council on Physical Fitness and Health, "Three miles of brisk walking will accomplish the same things as three miles of jogging. Our goal is to give more status to walking. Jogging has it, but we have to bring walking into its rightful place." That year, *Publishers Weekly* noted the release of no fewer than 14 books on the subject of walking, and a recently released report on fitness in America showed walking to be the nation's most popular form of exercise. She observed, "Capitalizing on this growing popularity the federal government is launching a national campaign to promote walking as a safe, painless way to fitness."[5]

Murphy argued that a sustained program of vigorous walking could do all the things that more demanding forms of exercise accomplished. That was what a study by Dr. Michael Pollack of Wake Forest University in North Carolina revealed in 1971. Pollack tested the effects of walking on body composition and cardiovascular function. Sixteen sedentary men aged 40 to 57 followed a 20-week walking program. Each man walked for around 40 minutes, four times a week, gradually increasing from 2.5 miles per session in 35.8 minutes to 3.2 miles in 41 minutes. By the end of the study, each of the subjects' heart rates had dropped by several points and all 16 had lost from two to three pounds, all of it fat. Their fitness gains were said to equal those obtained from a 30-minute, three-day-a-week jogging program.[6]

A 1981 article in a health-oriented magazine commented that some 35 million people in America walked daily but that "you might be tempted to say 'Walking is not really exercise, it's ... well, it's just walking.'" The fitness boom of the 1960s and 1970s, continued the article, led to an increased interest in vigorous sports such as tennis, skiing, and running, and they all became "in" sports. "Walking certainly doesn't have the charisma or the media popularity of these sports, but it shouldn't be overlooked as a route to fitness," observed the article. That boom in various sports benefited walking to a great extent as many people tried those sports but could not keep them up for various reasons (not in good enough shape, too expensive, lack of a suitable partner), yet their taste for exercise had been whetted and they looked around for an alternative. As walking required no special skills, no equipment, no baseline of fitness, and was safe, inexpensive, and not dependent on weather, it became a logical choice as an alternate exercise for many people.[7]

Charles Kuntzleman remarked in 1982 that physicians then were focusing more on preventive medicine than ever before. Since walking could be engaged in by people of varying ages and physical conditions it was an obvious choice for doctors to recommend walking as an exercise to their patients, and especially as study after study came out with reports of seemingly almost miraculous benefits. While Kuntzleman said there was no such thing as a perfect exercise, "yet walking comes very close. It's safe. Anyone can do it. It qualifies as an aerobic activity; and best of all, it slides easily into any daily routine." Going even further, he insisted vigorous walking produced the equivalent of a "runner's high." In his opinion, a walking session should last from a minimum of 20 minutes to a maximum of 60 minutes and take place at least three days a week, although four days would be better, with five or six days a week as the ultimate goal. Among the tips he gave for a person to build more walking into his day were the following, "Never drive less than one mile — walk instead," and "When it's practical, avoid elevators and escalators."[8] Later that same year, *Glamour* magazine enthused that more and more women were finding that walking to work was a painless way to squeeze exercise into a crowded day, "They find it helps them control their weight, gives them a good cardiovascular workout in addition to giving them a sense of overall well-being."[9]

Also in 1982, Lynn Langway wrote in *Newsweek* that more and more Americans were being involved in walking in some fashion with membership in hiking clubs having increased from coast to coast and even the awkward race-walking was said to be gaining ground. "Many of the proud new pedestrians are shin-splinted refuges from jogging who want a safer way to stay fit," she explained. According to the President's Council on Physical Fitness and Sports, about 36 million Americans over 18 walked almost every day for exercise — reportedly twice as many as 20 years earlier and more than six times the number that jog, "Nearly as many people walk to work as take public transportation."[10]

As the fad took hold, articles often became more confusing, more complicated, and more bizarre. Jean Maguire in 1983 penned a long article about how to turn everyday walking into a total fitness program. She provided a chart depicting eight separate "types" of walking (with a section on health benefits for each one). Those types were leisurely walking (an average speed of 1.0 to 2.0 miles per hour); mildly energetic walking (3.0 to 3.5); health walking (4.0 to 5.0); resistance walking, leg-lifting style (1.0 to 3.0, as in walking in sand at the beach); uphill climbing (1.0 to 2.0); weight-loaded walking (1.0 to 3.0, wearing a 20-lb backpack on city streets); walking while hiking (1.0 to 3.0); walking while pushing a baby carriage (1.0 to 3.0).[11]

Bill Gale reported in 1984 that experts did not promise greater longevity as a benefit from walking, yet went on to declare that "most people around the world who enjoy vigorous health at an advanced age are usually found to be great walkers." William Aikey, at one time Vermont's oldest resident, died in the 1970s aged 109. On his last birthday, he was asked reasons for his longevity, to which he replied, "Clean living and walking." Actor Greta Garbo was one of the world's most celebrated walkers and when Gale saw her striding along at age 78 "as fit and vigorous as a woman half her age," he concluded, "Walking may not actually increase your life span, but it obviously adds zest to the life you live."[12]

Other groups embraced walking and helped to spread the fad. In 1976, Weight Watchers International set out to develop a low intensity, long-duration exercise program for its members. Such a program had to be appropriate for anyone from 10 to 100 pounds overweight and it could not require special clothes or costly equipment. The choice ultimately was walking — a program called the Personal Exercise Plan, or Pepsteps. Members began with five minutes of callisthenics followed by 10 minutes of walking. By the 10th and last session of the program the walking component had increased to 55 minutes. Walking was also at that time the exercise of choice in the three Pritikin Longevity Centers where patients walked at least half an hour every day. Robert Sweetgall, author of *Fitness Walking*, said, "No one has discovered a fountain of youth, but a lifetime walking program will certainly slow the physiologic aging process." By this time, also, so-called power walking had become a minor craze of its own within the general category of walking as exercise. Power walkers attached weights to their waists, wrists, and ankles, with advanced power walkers adding weights totalling up to 20 percent of their body weight.[13]

According to American Sports Data, more than 50 million Americans walked for exercise at least once in 1985, compared with 33 million who jogged at least once. Reportedly, about 6,500 walking clubs promoted the activity. Several corporations, including Albertson's, Digital Equipment, Du Pont, and PepsiCo encouraged employees to walk for fitness.[14]

Srully Blotnick made the point in 1987 in *Forbes* about how many people were switching to walking from other more strenuous activities, usually because injuries had steered them away from some activity toward the relatively safer walking. Still, Blotnick thought one problem was that walkers were not as emotionally involved in their activity compared to, say, runners and joggers, who often kept logs of time and mileages and felt somewhat depressed if they hadn't run that day.[15]

Skye Wilson argued in 1988 that "health" and "high impact" had become a contradiction in terms and observed there were a lot less joggers and a lot less aerobics classes, while "Praised for its low impact fitness walking has taken off." Companies such as Kimberly-Clark and AT&T

sponsored power walking programs for their employees. Wilson said that, although many people dropped out of new exercise programs within a year, most fitness walkers stuck with their programs. One of the reasons for that difference, thought Wilson, was that walking programs held little chance of injuring the participants.[16]

Lilly Dickson, a registered nurse noted in 1989 the "huge revival" in walking, calling it the most popular form of exercise in Canada, with almost two-thirds of Canadians who exercised engaging in walking. Observing that walking had been abandoned over the previous century and that "Walking was passé—appropriate only for the old and poor," she said it was no coincidence that at the same time that walking lost its appeal, Canadians experienced a steady decline in health. Dickson also believed it was no coincidence that people who lived a long life were walkers, "They have much lower heart rates than inactive people.... A lower pulse means a longer life." The difference between a pulse of 80 and one of 70 was five million beats a year.[17]

Another piece of evidence that the fad of walking had arrived could be found in the pages of *Consumer Reports* in the February 1990 issue, wherein walking shoes were rated. According to the article, shoe manufacturing companies made 250 models of walking shoes and "Their ads often play up technology, making the shoes sound as complex as NASA's moon boots." A product like New Balance walking shoes had ads that claimed its products could accommodate "metatarsal head splay" (meaning the front of the shoe was roomy enough for the front of the foot to spread out, which it did when one was standing). One could also purchase walking shoes with "kinetic wedges," or air bladders, in the soles, or layers of foam impregnated with "microballoons" of nitrogen. Rated by the article were 13 men's and 13 women's models of walking shoes, most best sellers, ranging in price from $40 to $110. While the article did not say so directly, it reinforced the idea that walking shoes were distinct and unique [from "regular" walking shoes?] and probably necessarily so.[18]

With the craze in full bloom, *Good Housekeeping* published its "complete guide to walking" in the May 1992 issue, which involved "25 pages of walking tips, functional fashions, health and beauty help, nutritional know-how, fabulous food." However, most of those 25 pages had nothing much to do with walking. One page was an ad that featured all the advertisers that were in the walking special. Thirty products (along with photos) were listed, including Nair hair removal, Rogaine (a baldness treatment), and Crest toothpaste—products whose connection with walking was none too obvious.[19]

*Consumer Reports* was back with another rating of walking shoes in July 1993, this time of 32 models of walking shoes. Reportedly, more than

70 million Americans claimed they walked for exercise although, commented the publication, "sceptics suspect some of those millions are using the word 'exercise' loosely, walking is popular enough to have spawned a whole category of footwear — and sales of some $1.4 Billion last year. An activity isn't a sport, it seems, until it has its own shoe." Wondering whether special walking shoes were really necessary, the magazine took a somewhat more negative stance when it answered its own musing by saying, "Of course not. You can go for a walk in running shoes, aerobic shoes, or tennis shoes without worrying about the consequences. But for vigorous exercise, walking shoes work a little better."[20]

Journalist Mark Bricklin in 1995 cited a study done by doctors at Brown University School of Medicine that commented if just one out of every two adults began a regular walking program, $5.6 billion in medical care costs could be saved annually. And that was just in the heart disease area. National Walking Week was held that year from May 1–7. Bricklin argued that walking was becoming a born-again exercise, "No, not as part of our daily routine — that's gone forever — but as a special kind of supplement to our lifestyles, like vitamins, fiber and Comedy Central." Minority walking programs were said to be catching on in other cities, thanks to the Walking for Wellness program of the National Black Women's Health project. Oddly, he observed that thousands of people drove to their health clubs and there promptly went back outdoors to walk. Ellen Abbott, who instructed at the Boston Athletic Club and was the creative director of the Walk Reebok program, said she took 40 to 50 people outside ("the whole world is our gym") eight or nine times a week.[21]

From figures supplied by American Sports Data in 1996, more than 16 million people took two or more walks each week. Brisk walking (at a 15-minute per mile pace, fitness walking) was the most popular way to stay fit in the U.S. Kenneth Cooper, the man credited with inventing aerobics, even made changes in his own exercise program after conducting several walking studies at his Dallas-based facility, the Cooper Institute for Aerobics Research: "I became less concerned about getting my running in every night if I could get an appropriate amount of walking. I never would have considered that before.... I'm walking more than ever before — probably half walking and half running — and haven't lost anything as a runner."[22]

Another manifestation of the instrumental nature of walking in the modern craze era from 1979 onward, along with the involvement of more numbers and math equations, was the concept of calorie burn rates, burn totals, and weight loss. While they were mentioned pervasively in articles, they were almost always wrong, as they continuously confused people and led them astray. When a person walked a mile, he burned a specific number of calories (depending on body weight) and the number remained the same whether he walked that mile in 12 minutes, 20 minutes, or any other amount of time. Caloric burn rate per minute, of course varied with speed, but the burn total was always the same for a mile. An infrequent exception could occur if a person adopted, say, an exaggerated and unnatural arm movement at 12 minutes per mile that the person did not employ at 20 minutes per mile. But in the vast majority of cases, the simple law of physics applied: moving mass X through distance Y burned Z calories; speed was irrelevant. Running a mile produced the same general result. However, when the same man walked a mile in, say, 15 minutes, and a ran a mile in, say, eight minutes, the total calories burned was not the same because the methods of moving mass X (locomotion) were different (for example, in walking, at least one foot was always in contact with the ground, while in each step cycle in running there was always a brief moment when both feet were off the ground); running burned slightly more calories per mile than did walking.

Calories were burned by everybody all the time even when they were doing "nothing," including sleeping. On average it took about 15 calories per pound of body weight just for normal daily maintenance. Thus, a 140-pound person could consume 2,100 calories per day without experiencing any weight gain (about 90 calories burned per hour on average). In order to lose one pound of body weight it was necessary to burn 3,500 calories. Sleeping burned about 70 calories per hour, while talking when otherwise sedentary consumed 110 calories per hour.[23]

A 1979 article stated that brisk walking (four miles per hour) burned 400 calories an hour; regular walking (three miles per hour) burned 300 calories per hour; a window-shopping pace (two miles per hour) burned 200 calories per hour. Walking just one extra mile a day (15 minutes at a brisk pace), said the piece, would take off 10 pounds in one year. [Their math seemed to be 100 extra calories burned per day times 365 divided by the 3,500 needed to lose one pound, which roughly equalled 10 pounds.] The problem with this article and almost all that tackled the weight loss formulas was that the baseline was ignored; that is, the person walking 15 minutes a day that he did not do before had to give up some other activity. Assume it was a 140-pound person who reduced his time spent in a chair quietly reading by 15 minutes in order to walk, about 25 calories per 15 minutes. Therefore the extra calories burned would be 100 minus 25, which equalled a weight loss of 7.5 pounds per year, not 10.[24]

Later that year, Olympic runner Abby Hoffman wrote that an hour of brisk walking every other day could burn up about 4,800 calories per month, or almost 1.5 pounds. By her math, 15 hours of walking consumed

4,800 calories, or 320 per hour, or 80 per 15 minutes, which was significantly different from the above article that cited 100 per 15 minutes, although neither article mentioned a presumed weight for their example.[25]

Jane Brody, in the *New York Times* in 1980, said that on average a walk of three miles in an hour by a 160-pound person burned about 285 calories, and a 120-pound person would burn about 215 calories. If those 215 calories were burned up four times a week, said Brody, it could produce a 13-pound weight loss. Brody was another who forgot to subtract a baseline activity before computing weight loss.[26]

One of the farthest off the mark was an article in *Current Health 2* in 1981 that stated a major university recently found that jogging a mile in 8.5 minutes burned only 26 more calories than walking the same mile in 12 minutes. That study reportedly found that college students burned an average of 66 calories per mile while walking at three miles per hour but when they sped up to five miles per hour that increased to a burn rate of 124 calories per mile. That last claim was nonsense as it implied a breach in an elemental law of physics, although the first claim was accurate. A 150-pound person who walked briskly at 4.5 miles per hour burned 432 calories per hour (96 per mile) but when running at eight miles per hour, consumed 936 calories (117 per mile) an hour.[27]

Carol Krucoff, in the *Saturday Evening Post* in 1992, said a 150-pound person burned around 100 calories walking a mile and if that person took a brisk walk for 45 minutes (three miles) four times a week, he would lose 18 pounds. Krucoff also did not factor in a baseline activity. An article in 1993 in a different publication claimed that walking at 2.5 miles per hour burned 210 calories (84 calories per mile) while walking at 4.0 miles per hour burned 300 calories (75 per mile). Such results were also not compatible with the laws of physics.[28]

Even *Consumer Reports* (in 1993) calculated a weight loss out to nine pounds a year without taking into account the number of calories the person would have consumed doing something in lieu of walking. A couple of years later reporter Daryn Eller asserted that if a 100-pound woman walked three miles in an hour she burned 240 calories (80 per mile); at four miles per hour 350 (87.5); and at 4.5 miles per hour 440 (98). Kevin Knight argued in 1995 that one hour of brisk walking at five miles per hour burned 530 calories versus 480 for jogging [speed unspecified].[29]

So popular did walking become after the craze set in that this most natural of outdoor activities developed an indoor-walking subcategory. A brief mention was made in a 1983 article that if it was raining that was no excuse for not walking, because one could engage in indoor walking, at shopping malls and airports, for example.[30]

*Time* magazine ran a 1986 piece on the "growing breed of fitness faddists—the mall walkers." Most of them were said to be elderly. According to this article, more people were regular walkers than were runners, about 54 million compared to 34 million. Reporter Anastasia Toufexis commented that malls were conveniently located, climate controlled and security patrolled, and had rapidly emerged as the ideal site for stress-free walking. Said Helen Gulledge, 69, "We don't have to bother with dogs, traffic problems, rocks, hills or pollen." Shopping centers, eager to court potential shoppers when the retail outlets opened, were usually happy to open their doors before regular store hours. Some went so far as to measure off courses and issue walkers' maps. The quarter-mile circuit at the Northwoods mall in Peoria, Illinois, even included six stations for stretching and for light callisthenics. A pioneer in the field was the Ward Parkway Shopping Center of Kansas City. Reportedly, it had been welcoming mall walkers for 25 years [mostly, though, this was a fad that flourished in the 1980s] and actually opened its doors for three hours on holidays [this at a time when malls and their stores were closed on holidays] just to accommodate habitual walkers. "With local hospitals or health organizations," explained Toufexis, "the malls are also establishing walkers' clubs that offer T-shirts and buttons, merchant discounts, occasional free breakfasts and, most importantly, mileage logs for members." There was a group in Glendale, California, that called itself the Galleria Mall GoGetters. Maude Harris, 74, a member of the Georgia Square Strollers in Athens, Georgia, remarked, "We walk and we tell jokes and have a good clean fellowship." Toufexis concluded by noting, "Walkers keep as close tabs on their totals as runners do of their times."[31]

Mall walkers often got in at seven or eight o'clock in the morning, two to three hours before the shopping public, to walk along designated routes. Georgia Square started its program in 1985 and, said Kathy Kunzer, mall marketing director, "It has been a wonderful, widespread generator of goodwill for the mall, and a demonstrated health benefit and social inspiration for more than 200 participants." On any given day, 25 to 40 of those members would be in the mall walking before store hours; singly, in couples, or in groups. McDonald's always invited them to its "Happy Walker" center for coffee and to update their total walking mileages posted on a bulletin board. In the Georgia Square group women outnumbered men by a ratio of 60 to 40, with the age range being roughly 55 to 70.[32]

Robert Reinhold reported in the *New York Times*, also in 1986, that mall walking was a growing national phenomenon, especially in areas with harsh summers or winters, with thousands of people in Houston alone having discovered that the city's vast indoor shopping malls provided an excellent air-conditioned place to exercise, away from heat, humidity, dogs, motorists, and bugs. Reinhold said it all began a few years earlier, informally, but by the time he was writing many mall managements had embraced the trend as a public relations boon, with many malls then offering health-related incentives to attract more patrons. The Town and Country Center (Houston), for example, set up a hospital-affiliated walkers' club that provided members with a stop-smoking clinic and exercise classes, along with store discounts. According to Juli Bump, Town and Country marketing director, "The merchants love it. This is good community public relations." About one year earlier, Town and Country set up a walkers' club in collaboration with Spring Branch Memorial Hospital as part of the hospital's cardiac program. By 1986 the club had 1,300 members who had collectively registered 16,600 mall miles in the preceding 15 or so months. (Jogging or running was forbidden in the mall as, supposedly, it led to an undue insurance liability risk.) The 145-store mall had set aside a vacant store on the third level as "walk-a-mall" headquarters for fitness classes, exercises, and medical exams. Members received a free T-shirt after 100 miles, and other gifts when they reached the 500- and 1,000-mile marks. Douglas and Helen Brown of Cincinnati said, "Wherever we go, we find a mall. It's much more comfortable than outdoors. There are no hills, and we can set our own pace and keep it."[33]

A couple of years later, journalist William Stockton stated no one knew how many mall walkers there were but that their total was believed to be "substantial," usually made up of older people. "The mall walkers are attracted by a large space heated in the winter and cooled in the summer, where there is no traffic, where the surface is smooth and conducive to walking and where there are no fears about safety," he explained. Denver heart surgeon Marvin Pomerantz remarked, "Many of my patients can find lots of reasons not to walk: it's too hot or too cold or too much traffic, or it's dangerous." He told them to drive to the nearest mall and start walking.[34]

Avia Athletic Footwear, a division of footwear maker Reebok, estimated in 1989 there could be as many as 500,000 mall walkers in America. To capitalize on that market, Avia had just introduced a walking shoe designed "to give extra traction for smoother, slicker mall floors" and "to propel the body's momentum forward." Some scorned the mall walking trend. Bradford Ketchum, editor of *The Walking Magazine* (who regularly walked the two miles from his home to his office in downtown Boston), said, "I like the fresh air and trees, the song of a bird or the smell of flowers, a little wind on your back, and the surprise of suddenly coming upon a lake in the woods. In a mall you're likely to turn a corner and discover an

Orange Julius." John Robinson, a sociologist at the University of Maryland, disliked the thought of exercising in "the typically sterile atmosphere" of a shopping center. He said it brought to mind the cult movie *The Night of the Living Dead* in which an army of zombies roamed aimlessly through malls. Some malls were said even to have asked walkers what type of music they preferred but, remarked reporter Joseph Pereira, "mall walkers aren't fussy. In fact, they actually seem to like the stuff piped out over the loudspeakers." Even mall walkathons were starting to be held. One month earlier, animal rights advocates had raised $2,500 walking 23 laps — about 12 miles — at Fairfield Mall in Chicopee, Massachusetts. Woodfield Shopping Mall in Schaumburg, Illinois, launched major center events with a mall-walking contest. Contestants were asked to dress in orange, the mall's color, and winners (those who logged the most miles) got gift certificates for use at mall stores. Joseph Piombino, who did six miles a day at Woodfield, got a $50 certificate after logging 3,000 miles in one contest. "I've walked across America," he said, "and I did it at Woodfield Shopping Mall." At least one college offered a semester-long course in mall walking. Contra Costa Community College in Richmond, California, conducted classes at a local mall and graded students on attendance and willpower.[35]

The Suburban Hospital in Bethesda, Maryland, sponsored an early morning, free indoor walking program at a local mall. Hospital staff members were available to monitor members' progress, take blood pressure, and give tips on fitness. At the end of 1990, Bradford Ketchum estimated that more than one million Americans — the majority over the age of 50 — got their walking exercise in malls. After this period, media interest in mall walking faded away and the activity received next to no attention from the media. Whether it faded away in popularity among its adherents to the same extent is unclear.[36]

With walking as exercise becoming such a fad in the 1980s — with many books and articles on the subject, in addition to participants — came the marketing of other items in connection with walking as manufacturers fought it out with each other in the marketplace to sell walking items for which there had been no demand and for which there was no need. They were very successful.

# 11
# Marketers Target Walking

> *"Some industry analysts wonder whether walkers will buy special walking shoes that offer few advantages over wing tips or loafers or sneakers — which people buy, when you stop and think about it, for walking."*
> Forbes, 1986.
>
> *"But can it [walking] be turned into a sport, complete with a full-fledged marketing mechanism? And if so, is it just a case of P. T. ('sucker born every minute') Barnum redux?"*
> Carol Hall, 1986.
>
> *"... walking shoes conveniently lower the standards of exercise to include an activity that was too easy to be called exercise in the past."*
> Steven Barnett, 1987.

Reporter Mary Pinkham observed in 1983 that for around $70 one could buy a Jogger Mate Pulse Meter into which one inserted the little finger, with a moving needle register on the device producing a pulse reading. The meter made it much easier to determine if one's pulse was indeed in the target zone area.[1]

Raben Publishing came out in May 1986 with *The Walking Magazine*, the first such publication of its kind. Raben claimed its audience could be one out of every two Americans. It based that claim on statistics that showed walking was a sport engaged in by about 70 million adults for recreation, and an additional 27 million more for strenuous aerobic exercise. One of Raben's hopes was that its advertisers would include those firms that manufactured "walking" shoes, then about 10 in number. Judging by the number of walking shoes on the market, remarked Raben vice president of marketing, Rich Powers, the magazine would benefit because "Marketers saw this as an opportunity not to get left behind like they did with the aerobic craze." Launched as a quarterly magazine for its first year (at $2.95 per issue) it was set to publish monthly thereafter.[2]

From the beginning, of course, shoe manufacturers led other specialty items such as apparel, socks, and accessories in pitching to walking enthusiasts, especially, said business reporter Judann Dagnoli, as "Ads promote walking as a panacea for everything from heart disease to osteoporosis." The walking shoe was once considered a geriatric or orthopaedic aid produced by specialty companies and was struggling to overcome that stodgy image as major athletic-shoe manufacturers entered that market segment. Some of those companies were enthusiastic about the prospects (with 55 million Americans said to walk for exercise), estimating walking shoes could be a $100 million market in three years. Others were less enthusiastic, such as Puma, which did sell walking shoes but was not prepared to risk large sums of money on them in advertising support. Enthusiastic or not, all the makers were involved as none wanted to be left out or to miss the boat. Market leader Rockport was then modernizing its lines with new colors and styles. Reportedly there were then 30 makers of walking shoes marketing at least 80 styles (a "flood" of new entries were said to have all arrived in the first half of 1986). Blurring the lines of the walking-shoe segment had been the entry of athletic-shoe manufacturers such as Converse, Nike, and Reebok. "Everything from summer sandals to hiking boots are being positioned as walking shoes," remarked Dagnoli.[3]

Manufacturers were said to define the true walking shoe as a technically advanced product, providing such features as a "toe box" with extra room, less shock absorption in the heel than running shoes, a more flexible curved sole to facilitate a rocking motion, and perhaps extra-absorbent fabric or lining. At the time, Puma sold three walking-shoe styles but was waiting for solid evidence of a developing market before putting up big ad dollars. Only one print ad, costing around $12,000, had supported the Puma line, said Joseph Grimaldi, vice president at Puma's ad agency Mullen Advertising. "It's an inconsequential category," he said. "We sell 140 different types of shoes. We've got other opportunities to exploit." Dagnoli added, "Most walking-shoe marketers agree that interest in the product has been generated by the media and that it must be aggressively cultivated to create consumer demand." At Rockport, the firm's advertising had focused more on the fitness benefits of walking than on its expensive ProWalkers shoe. However, Rockport marketing vice president Beverly Daane declared that was changing because "We're tired of educating the public so that the competition can take over the market." One Nike walking shoe, the Healthwalker, featured ads with the line, "Stop your husband from becoming an old man." Ad copy claimed that walking could prevent osteoporosis: "It helps bone tissue renew itself, literally reversing the aging process." One unnamed research company analyst said, "I'm not sure to what degree a walking shoe is very necessary."[4]

Briefly tracing the history of walking shoes, Lewis Spalding said a maker of high-end, brand-name men's shoes had been offering designated walkers for men for over a century and for women for nearly as long, while one athletic-shoe maker had carried both women's and men's walkers in its line since 1948. But around 1983 and 1984, the market for walking shoes suddenly exploded, attracting both fitness enthusiasts (transferring over from the more hazardous running) and more sedentary strollers. Serving that demand early and with special intensity was manufacturer Rockport. Further impetus was given when L. L. Bean devoted feature space to Vasque (Red Wing, Minnesota) walkers for women and men in its Fall 1985 catalog. At first the upsurge in demand for walkers came mainly from men but soon switched to women with the latter outbuying men by a margin of three to one nationwide by 1986.[5]

According to Spalding, the walking shoe's market potential was about 25.6 million women and 15.9 million men, a total that came from a 1986 survey of the National Sporting Goods Association (NSGA). A prediction from NSGA was that walking shoes would experience a 1986–1987 boom comparable to that enjoyed by aerobics equipment whose sales went up 229 percent from 1984 to 1985. They also felt the main sales target age to be 35 to 55, but NSGA did admit "definitions of shoe types are not precise, nor are the qualifications for a man or a woman to be termed a walker." In one of the biggest volume family shoe stores in the Southeast — the 24,000 square foot Tops in Asheville, North Carolina — owner Robert Carr exclaimed, "Walking shoes are selling through so fast here we can't even assemble enough to back up an ad. I compliment the manufacturers for the way they've made not just the public, but doctors as well, all conscious of this fresh category in footwear.... I've never seen any idea translate into sales floor action as fast."[6]

Late in 1986 an article on walking in *Fortune* magazine mused, "Some industry analysts wonder whether walkers will buy special walking shoes that offer few advantages over wing tips or loafers or sneakers—which people buy, when you stop and think about it, for walking."[7]

Around the same time, business reporter Carol Hall asked rhetorically, "Will marketers be able to convince consumers that they need special equipment to do something that they do as naturally as eating or sleeping." As recently as five years earlier, she said, the walking shoe failed as a fad. Nike, for example, launched the Pathfinder model around 1979, hoping to catch some of its running-shoe customers who had slowed down to a walk. Sales were disappointing, however, and the shoe was phased out a few years later. Neither did *Walking! Journal*, launched in 1983 by Orenda Media, get off the ground. But figures from American Sports Data convinced many the time had come. Eighty-four million Americans were said to have walked for fun at least once in 1985; 40 million participated at least once in brisk "aerobic" walking; 20 million went on brisk walks an average of once a week; and 1.9 million totalled at least 1,500 briskly walked miles each. The Sporting Goods Manufacturers Association did not bother tracking walking-shoe sales as a separate category until 1986. In the first quarter of that year, walking shoes sold 1.4 million pairs (priced from $40 to $100) with retail sales totaling $36.6 million. For the same period, running shoes sold three million pairs for a retail sales total of $86.1 million. Overall, the athletic shoe market was one of $8 billion annually.[8]

Richard Polk owned a group of Colorado-based stores known as the Pedestrian Shops that sold walking shoes and paraphernalia such as walking guide books, walking sticks, walking shorts, and pedometers. He said, "I believe the potential market for it is much larger than it was for running. Also, the life cycle of the market is potentially much longer. You can do it 'til you drop and, if we're right about [its health benefits], you can drop a little later." Two walking magazines then were being published; *Walkways* had joined *The Walking Magazine*. That latter publication had a circulation of 500,000 after its fourth issue, having launched with a guaranteed circulation of 300,000 for its first issue. In addition to selling ad space to walking-shoe manufacturers, it also had advertisers like General Foods (cereals), Sanka decaffeinated coffee, Casio televisions, MacGregor tennis rackets, and Maserati cars.[9]

Hall reported the number of fitness walkers was expected to grow to between 80 and 90 million by 1990. (Hall defined a fitness walker as one who moved at speeds of from 2.5 to 5.0 miles per hour.) The number of walking events grew from 2,500 in 1985 to 10,000 in 1986, while the number of running marathons, in contrast, declined 38 percent between 1980 and 1985. According to a Gallup Poll, the number of people who defined themselves as joggers dropped from 18 percent of the respondent sample in 1984 to 15 percent in 1985. Said Beverly Daane, Rockport vice president of marketing, "People are not so much into the burning pain of running." A couple of years earlier, Nike reported its market research showed that 60 percent of its running shoes were being bought for uses other than running. Shoe comfort was in. By the time of Hall's article over 100 shoe makers had reportedly launched casual walking shoes and at least 25 of those had marketed shoes for the fitness walker.[10]

In Hall's opinion, the marketing challenge was to convince consumers that their sneakers, loafers, or even old running shoes were not appropriate for distance walking: "Marketers have already gotten behind the concept with lines emphasizing the 'biochemical' needs of feet and legs." The most common design feature that then distinguished a walking shoe as such, she thought, was a lower midsole than found on a running shoe, and more padding on the inside with less on the outside. Athletic-shoe maker Reebok purchased the Rockport firm in the fall of 1986 as consolidation within the industry took place. Nike spokeswoman Mary Marckx commented, "We consider walking one of our important programs for the coming year. Our feeling is, physical fitness as a part of life in America is here to stay, and we see walking as an important part of this." With respect to walking Hall believed there was little doubt it would be taken up by more and more people although she cynically wondered, "But can it be turned into a sport, complete with a full-fledged marketing mechanism? And if so, is it just a case of P. T. ('sucker born every minute) Barnum redux?" Matt Zale, president of U.S. Marathon Limited (a national marketer of athletic footwear) replied to that point by remarking, "To be honest with you, there's a little bit of hype in it. People don't need [walking shoes], people don't need running shoes, tennis shoes, whatever." To which Hall added, "Manufacturers just did a good job of making consumers think they needed different footwear for every activity. And U.S. consumers do have a penchant for gear. All agree that once shoppers decide they are 'into' a sport, they get a yen for any and all equipment that goes with it."[11]

Early in 1987, journalist William Geist did an article on walking paraphernalia that was both cynical and a little tongue-in-cheek. Expensive walking shoes, he observed, were sometimes called "walking systems." A new store had just opened in New York City called the Urban Hiker, which described itself as "America's First Walking Store." It was a store for people the owner called "serious walkers." Besides stocking dozens of walking shoes (priced from $45 to $135) and "complete" walking outfits ($60 to $165), the outlet sold walking accessories such as imported high-tech walking "poles" made of ultralight steel that telescoped down to briefcase size. While Geist was in the store, a customer, Marshall Lieber, dropped in to ask if the shop carried "walking underpants." It did. Lieber already owned ProWalker walking shoes, a walking shirt, walking shorts, a walking sweat suit, and walking socks. (The Rockport Walking Sock had a padded heel, bulbous toe, and retailed for $7.50.) Additionally there were walking hats and walking gloves available.[12]

How did all that walking gear differ from, for example, jogging outfits, wondered Geist? Store owner George Pakradoonian, Jr., replied, "In subtle ways. Walking suits have maybe a little more style to them, perhaps, because, like, you might want to go in some place" [such as a store]. One of the store's customers was David Balboa, whose business card read, "The Walking Psychotherapist, M.S.W., C.S.W., M.B.A." He stated that he had developed a psychotherapeutic walking technique that combined racewalking with the Brazilian Samba. Store manager Raymond Rosario gave instruction in the shop on how to walk. Among the books and magazines sold there was The *Walking Book*, with chapter titles such as "Meet Your Feet" and instructions in how to walk. An ad in *The Walking Magazine* was for a book titled *Walk, Don't Die*, which "shows you how jogging kills, callisthenics cripple, diets debilitate and aerobics disable." Owner Pakradoonian had been working at his father's shoe store when he got the idea to open the walking store. "My father thought I was absolutely nuts," he admitted. The father added, "Everybody walks! Why do you need a store to take a walk?" Pakradoonian denied the term "walking shoe" was redundant, although Geist observed that passers-by [and he] tended to heap scorn on the concept. Herb Vincent was one who passed the new store. He told Geist "that he did not feel the need for a $165 Gore-Tex walking outfit and $100 Vibram-soled shoes 'to take a &*%?x walk.'"[13]

Upon viewing *The Walking Magazine*, comedian Jay Leno reportedly quipped that Barnum was right — there was a sucker born every minute. What new information, he wondered, "could this magazine possibly contain?" Reporter Susanna Levin noted that Leno was not the only one to point out that most of us have been walking since we were two. What, all of a sudden, was new about walking? "In truth, not much," she declared.[14]

Actress Rita Moreno marched through New York City's Central Park in May 1987 to publicize National Walking Week. (She was a sort of ambassador-at-large, and enthused, "Signs of the walking boom are everywhere.... Walking has gone from a phenomenon to a trend. No—more than a trend. It's a fad." In recent weeks New York journalists had received piles of walking-related data from public relations firms that were trying to "put the walking boom on a sound statistical footing," as one publicity agent said. One of those was the Dr. Scholl's Walking Study that claimed nurses (5.3 miles per day) and security guards (4.2 miles) walked the most on the job. Reporter Glenn Collins observed, "But walking, it seems, is not simply walking. There are in fact 26 different kinds of walking, from hiking to strolling to racewalking, according to the Walkways Center in Washington." One of Walking Week's partners, Sanka, was also promoting a line of National Walking Week greeting cards.[15]

One of the longer articles to look at the marketing craze, as well as other aspects of walking, was by Kerry Pechter in the summer of 1987 in the business publication *Across the Board*. At a January 1987 press conference by shoe manufacturer Reebok, waiters wore T-shirts that read "No thanks, I'll Walk" as the manufacturer announced it would soon launch four new shoes designed specifically for walking. Overall, Reebok and its affiliates (it had just acquired Rockport) were expected to introduce more than two dozen models of walking shoes in 1987. According to Harvey Lauer, a market researcher who specialized in sports trends, about 130 firms would field new or existing walking shoes that year. While the entire U.S. shoe market was $22 billion annually, estimates for walking shoe sales ranged from $200 million to $1 billion a year. Major shoe manufacturers clearly saw a big trend still gaining momentum. Data from the National Sporting Goods Association asserted that over 50 million Americans described themselves as regular walkers. To Pechter they were an odd assortment ranging from serious to casual: lunch-hour strollers, day hikers, racewalkers, power walkers, and mall walkers. "The mere act of putting one foot in front of the other seems to have become a sport," concluded Pechter.[16]

Texas-based American Volksport Association led 300,000 people on organized walks in 1986, while Walkabout International in San Diego organized over 1,400 walks a year in that city alone. Pechter thought the walking boom did not appear to be a single metamorphosis of the jogging boom, but "It is a related phenomenon with a separate and highly segmented market. In fact, Reebok's press conference in January heralded not a new trend but the last phase of the fitness boom that started back in the mid-'70s." Kevin Brown, Nike's director of corporate communications, declared "The whole phenomenon is people who haven't exercised in an organized fashion since they left school."[17]

Pechter then detailed some of the earlier days of the walking boom. First company to enter the walking shoe market was Rockport, a Marlboro, Massachusetts, firm whose success with a $55 walking shoe called Rocsport was said to have provided the initial spark. Founded in 1972 by Bruce Katz, Rockport began as a maker of casual street shoes. In 1979, Katz became intrigued by the lightness and shock absorption of running shoes and decided to build those features into a casual shoe. The shoe caught on and Rockport revenues jumped dramatically from $7.1 million in 1980 to $95.5 million in 1986. Katz said his walking shoe provided a rallying point. There was a core group of people interested in walking and Rockport tapped into that. "We talked to them and created events. In so doing, we started a snowball effect that started gathering momentum over the last 18 months and is now really gaining speed," he explained. "We put millions of dollars and several years of effort into this, and, lo and behold, we have a movement." Rockport was purchased in 1986 by Reebok for $118 million. However, many believed Rockport's success alone had not been enough to trigger the boom. For one thing, Rockport was building a casual shoe with walking technology, a very different shoe from the 1986 jogging-style walking shoes, which were far and away the most popular. Harvey Lauer observed, "Rockport's success didn't have much to do with walking. But Rockport's promotions may have stirred the pot a little."[18]

Psychologist Lauer, after taking up jogging, set up American Sports Data, Inc., in Hartsdale, New York, to study the characteristics of the purchasers of running shoes. In 1984 he added the walking market and sold his data to clients such as Nike, Adidas, *Sports Illustrated*, and *The Walking Magazine*. "I was the first in the research field to recognize walking. I measured aerobic walking as early as 1984," he said. The typical walker in 1987, said Lauer, was a woman of middle age; 60 percent of walkers were women and 38 percent of walkers were over the age of 55. According to Lauer, the walking market was not composed of joggers who had switched to a less bone-jarring sport. "That's one of the myths the media have created," he argued. "Walkers aren't burned-out joggers, they're not injured runners. I did a pretest, and out of the first 100 walkers, only two or three said they began walking when they stopped running." NPD Research, a Long Island market research group, reported that one in three runners were between 18 and 34 years old, while one-third of all walking shoe purchasers were over 55. One in three joggers earned $40,000 or more a year, but fewer than one in five walkers earned that much. Lauer's latest data, based on a survey of more than 17,000 people across the country, found that 123 million Americans—70 percent of adults—walked at least once in 1986 for either exercise or recreation.[19]

By Lauer's definition, 25 million people qualified as "exercise walkers," people who did it year-round, or seasonally, and walked a minimum of two miles a week. Of those, he thought, 15 million or so were "remote prospects" for buying a shoe designed specifically for exercise walking, leaving only around five to 10 million as likely purchasers. He believed eight percent of the walking population were essentially dog walkers and 20 percent were what he called functional walkers—that is, people who lived in, say, Scarsdale and walked 1.5 miles to the train station. Forty-five percent of all walkers started because they wanted to lose weight, and 12 percent were "old guys" who took up walking as therapy for a heart problem. According to Lauer, 25 percent of the walking population moved at a normal pace; 61 percent walked somewhat faster than normal; and 14 percent moved at a much faster than ordinary pace.[20]

In explaining the walking boom, Lauer stated that walkers were not the vanguard of a new trend, but the stragglers of the last one—"they're bringing up the rear of the fitness boom." Running was the spearhead, the sport that launched the fitness boom. It paved the way for the rise of the more vigorous second-phase activities such as aerobic dancing. A third stage of the revolution started in the mid 1980s, Lauer continued: "We began to see lots of people who were formerly sedentary emulators of the fitness lifestyle, people who did nothing, who may have been overweight or smoked, but who liked the idea of fitness and wore $150 velour running suits and headbands while they stood around smoking." Those people found there were several less taxing, easier activities they could participate in such as soft aerobics, where one foot never left the ground, and fitness walking. "It is by nature less demanding than running, and lots of people who were reticent about running are now trying this, as one of the third-generation sports," said Lauer.[21]

Steven Barnett, cultural anthropologist and marketing consultant, saw three dynamics at work in the walking boom. One was that of adults seeking softer forms of exercise than jogging; a second was that many people fell under the spell of what he called "contagious magic," that is, an unconscious belief that simply wearing athletic shoes would somehow turn them into athletes. "Third, walking shoes conveniently lower the standards of exercise to include an activity that was too easy to be called exercise in the past." When people bought walking shoes, said Barnett, "it gives them the illusion of exercise, if not the reality. With walking shoes, you can still have it in your mind that you are committed and involved in exercise." He added, "Four or five years ago, wearing walking shoes would not have conveyed a set of health-oriented values. But today it does. A lot of the attraction of walking shoes is related to a redefinition of exercise."[22]

Nike had introduced a walking shoe in 1979, the same year as Rockport. That shoe, said to be popular but not profitable, was dropped in 1984, but in 1987 the firm had a line of four new walking shoes. Virtually all of the major running-shoe firms—Nike, Saucony, Brooks, Adidas, Converse, Puma, and others—had walking shoes in stores or at least on the drawing board, as did most of the traditional shoe companies. For Nike, walking shoes represented replacement business for the decline in sales of running shoes to non-joggers (for fashion). For others, it was new business. Brooks, a small company in Rockford, Michigan, initially used the cheapest method of retooling, said Pechter, "it simply repositioned its running shoe as a walking shoe, on the basis of testimonials by podiatrists." Adidas made walking shoes, javelin-throwing shoes, parachuting shoes, windsurfing shoes, bobsledding shoes, and fencing shoes, among others. Pechter commented that much of the advertising for walking shoes was directed at consumer uncertainty over the need for a "technical" walking shoe. "Walking is simple. The equipment shouldn't be," proclaimed one ad. "Yes, you really do need special shoes for walking," said another.[23]

With respect to the boom in sales of walking shoes, Lauer remarked, "This is the first time in the history of the industry that the manufacturers have attempted to foist a product from above onto a sports population without first responding to consumer demand." A marketer at one of the major athletic shoe firms agreed: "With aerobics and jogging the consumers started the fad first and the publishers and the shoe companies followed them. But this is total hype."[24]

Many walking events in the previous few years had been staged and promoted by shoe companies. In 1984, Rockport funded a year-long 11,208-mile solo walk and lecture tour through all 50 states by a walking enthusiast named Rob Sweetgall and sponsored a film of the journey called *Walk, America!* Since 1984 Rockport has sponsored walks in more than a dozen cities, involving an estimated 50,000 participants. Membership in the Saucony Walking Club came automatically to Saucony customers. Puma product manager Paul Oparowski said his firm was organizing a club and walking events. Rockport sent the names and addresses of 200,000 of its shoe customers to *The Walking Magazine*, which sent them direct-mail material. Reebok, Saucony, Nike, and Rockport had all offered their buyers free subscriptions to the magazine, which in turn had assisted Rockport in staging events. *Prevention* magazine, whose subscriber demographics matched those of people in the walking boom, started a walking club among its readers a year earlier. Some 75,000 of that magazine's three million subscribers had paid to join the club, and *Prevention* offered advertisers special access to those members through the cosponsorship of such events as "Walk Your Dog Month," a venture in conjunction with pet-food maker Ralston-Purina.[25]

Rockport's Bruce Katz argued that publicity alone could not have created a walking movement if there had not been a lot of interest in walking to begin with. Katz saw a groundswell of enthusiasm for walking and believed that younger people were becoming more interested. Walkways Center in Washington, D. C., a nonprofit walking organization (a sort of clearinghouse) that had spun off from a walking-products catalog in 1985, had 4,000 paid members nationwide. To reach their peak, walking shoes would have to become a fashion item, not merely a fitness item. "For every gung-ho walker who laces up at dawn for a five-mile hike, there will have to be five other people wearing walking shoes to the supermarket or for puttering around the yard," declared Pechter. Lauer believed walking shoes had a number of obstacles to overcome to reach that peak. One was that there were no male walking heroes, at least not among the living. Walking shoes lacked the endorsement of a role model like Larry Bird (basketball shoes) or John McEnroe (tennis shoes). "Women have more common sense, and they recognize the benefits of walking immediately," said one shoe marketer. "Men won't try something new until they're sure that it's macho."[26]

At General Nutrition Centers (GNC) the company tried to reach their existing and potential customers through "lifestyle marketing." A study of their market research department in 1986 revealed that their typical customers were heavy vitamin users, 50 or older, active, upscale socially and economically, and activist when it came to health. Tim Megyesy, GNC director of marketing, said, "Our customer profile coincided with that of fitness walking enthusiasts. To capitalize on this match, we decided to have GNC positioned as the location for fitness walking information and products." They expected to see an increase in fitness walking popularity due to the aging of America's population. The University of Maryland's Survey on American Recreational Trends revealed that more than half of the population between 45 and 64 years of age, and 41 percent of those 65 and older, walked for pleasure and health.[27]

Having decided to position their 1,150 stores (900 of which were in malls) as "the home of fitness walking," said Megyesy, GNC hired an outside firm to develop a "multiphase lifestyle marketing plan." The first phase began in August 1987 and involved offering "America's Fitness Walking" kit for $19.95. The kit included a pedometer, sun visor, coupon book, fitness walking handbook, vitamins, a sample issue of the *Walking Magazine*, and other items. To encourage repeat visits to their stores, GNC launched their "America's Fitness Walking Challenge." For each 15 miles walked, a customer could go back to the store, show his pedometer to the clerk for verification, and receive an envelope to order a state pin, offered free except for postage and handling. Within each store was a three-foot section identified as the fitness walking area. It displayed pedometers, weights for walking, fitness walking books, and other items for sale, and posted notices of various walking clubs' events. In eight weeks GNC sold over 10,000 fitness walking kits.[28]

*Prevention* presented a list of gadgets and walking paraphernalia in its June 1992 issue. Included in the list were reflective vests; a cool-down towel for $19.95 (a Gore-Tex pocket filled with ice cubes); a walk bottle; lifelights fanny pack with reflective tape (the lights used batteries), a pedometer for $29.95, a pedometer for $39.95 (this one counted calories burned, told time, and sounded an alarm when the wearer had met his workout goal), and a combination personal stereo and pedometer for $59.95 (a cassette player with an AM/FM radio that also counted the wearer's steps and sounded a beep when time was up). The *Prevention* Walking Club offered its members T-shirts and sweatshirts with reflective ink front and back (priced at $15 and $20), and a one-inch 14-carat, gold walker's charm that could be worn on a bracelet or neck chain, described by the publication as follows: "Your personal walking icon says to the world, 'I'm a walker.'"[29]

In 2001 it was reported that American consumers were taking up the Japanese fad for electronic pedometers, with sales in America reportedly soaring. In Japan, the interest in pedometers was sparked by a movement called 10,000 Steps a Day, which promised that better health and slimmer waists resulted from walking that many steps a day. Reporter Ian Austen tested four different models. All converted the steps counted into miles or kilometers, and two of the units calculated how many calories the walking had burned. However, when it came to converting strides into distance, said Austen, accuracy declined. All the pedometers required the owner to measure his stride length and enter it into the unit. It was not as simple an operation as it appeared. One of the units suggested a person walk 100 or 200 feet, count how many steps there were, and divide. Austen found that no method was perfect, as hills often shortened stride length, while moving a little faster often lengthened the step. David R. Bassett, Jr., professor of exercise science and sports management at the University of Tennessee at Knoxville had worn a pedometer for a research project, from the time he got up until he went to bed, for an entire year. His average over that time was 9,500 steps a day. As to the 10,000 steps-per-day program, Bassett commented, "To me this is almost a case where promotion of a physical activity has gotten ahead of science. We don't have rock-hard data showing that walking 10,000 steps is beneficial."[30]

According to a 2000 report, inventor Trevor Baylis of the UK had figured out how to harness the energy generated by walking. His latest device, which had just been registered at the patent office, would be worn in the shoe and power a mobile phone or palmtop computer as its user walked.[31]

While most experiments and studies involving walking concentrated on health and medical effects, some delved into the psychological aspects of walking. Those efforts ranged from serious academic studies to pop psychology reports.

# 12
# Psychological Aspects of Walking

*"A person who has straightened out her walk has straightened out her life."*
*Mademoiselle*, 1979.

*"If we shuffle along we see ourselves walking as if we felt down, and we decide that we must, therefore, feel down."*
Sara Snodgrass, 1987.

*"[The way we walk] is a silent flag that reveals the intricacies of our inner lives. Our walk is like a second signature."*
Helen Fisher, 1989.

Mostly, studies on psychological aspects of walking were a modern phenomenon, from the late 1970s onward. However, a few earlier reports had appeared. A 1915 news account noted that an unnamed Pittsburgh professor had invented a machine for recording the human gait. According to the professor, a person could be identified by his manner of walking as easily as by his fingerprints. From a person's gait certain personality characteristics could be inferred, he insisted: "The man with the dragging gait is the man without a heart"; "The woman who has difficulty in lifting her heels from the ground when she walks is a whiner"; "The woman with the dragging gait is the woman without spine"; and "The man with the snappy step has plenty of pep."[1]

James Cutting and Lynn Kozlowski, both of Wesleyan University in Connecticut, videotaped six college students in 1978 as they walked back and forth. The men and women had normal gaits and were about the same size. Patches of reflecting material were wrapped around the subjects' joints and taped to their hips and shoulders. At high contrast and low brightness settings, the walkers appeared as clusters of bright dots moving across a television screen. All familiarity cues such as clothing and hairstyles were obliterated. Two months later the walkers (who knew each other) viewed the videotapes and tried to identify the walkers. They guessed correctly 38 percent of the time (chance was 16.7 percent), but were no more accurate at recognizing themselves than they were at identifying the others. Although no feedback was given, the viewers improved with practice; they averaged 27 percent accuracy on the first three trials but moved up to 49 percent on the final three trials. Viewers reported that speed, bounciness, and rhythm were valuable clues to the identity of walkers with length of stride and arm swing also being helpful.[2]

An example of a pop psychology piece could be found in the unsigned article that appeared in the July 1979 issue of *Mademoiselle*, wherein it was declared in the subhead, "The way you walk, like the way you write, is a personality indicator and a valid way of analyzing who you are. A person who has straightened out her walk has straightened out her life." Defined were several types of walks. In the "sexy walk" there was a calculated up-and-down hip motion and a thrusting of the chest, "You keep your arms close to your body so other people are aware of your body, too. You like to be the center of attention." Movement incorporating an elevated ribcage and an abrupt arm swing were indicative of the "brisk" walk, and that meant, "You're not quite the success you want to be yet, but you're up-and-coming." According to the article, it should be possible to cure personality defects by altering the manner of walking. Psychologist Joyce Brothers agreed: "You can change the way you perceive yourself, the way other people perceive you, by changing your walk."

Kinesiologist Maurita Robarge remarked that a person's walk "varies according to the situation," that is, if a person was outgoing then their walk would be also. But if a person was both outgoing and depressed, the gait would reflect that. "Chances are you'll cheer up if you force your walk to," advised *Mademoiselle*. Analyzing other gaits, the article stated, "If your arms swing easily from the shoulder, you have confidence to spare. If you don't have much arm swing, you'd rather be inconspicuous. If you don't have much leg swing, you're shy. You are capable — not on the make — if you swivel or rotate your hips a bit when you push a leg forward." Then the article described the walking style associated with each of the 12 astrological signs; for example, Aries (March 21 to April 20), "Your walk is an energetic march or very prancy. You lean forward leading with you head, too impatient to wait for the rest of your body," and Cancer (June 21 to July 20), "Your walk is a kind of stroll and you tend to a sideways gait, often bumping your shoulder against your companion."[3]

Psychology researchers set up two tables in Manhattan in 1981 for passing pedestrians to stop—187 did—and write down their thoughts, what they had on their minds while they walked. One table was uptown near Tiffany's at the fashionable intersection of Fifth Avenue and 57th Street. Thoughts most commonly reported there had to do with the "immediate environment" and most were upbeat, how great it was to be in New York City, and so forth. Next in frequency of occurrence were thoughts about "work," followed by "love." The second table was located downtown in Union Square, a down-at-the-heels shopping area near Greenwich Village. Leading the list of thoughts there were "shopping" and "money," next came thoughts the researchers classified as "future plans," then came "love." Results also showed that virtually no one thought about politics. Thoughts of more than half the respondents were classified by the researchers as dealing with the present, 34 percent as dealing with the future, and 10 percent as dealing with the past.[4]

Later that year, *Glamour* published a pop psychology piece that declared, "You may not realize it, but the way you walk says a lot about you. It can tell others whether you feel assertive or timid, are in a relaxed mood or tense, approachable or standoffish;" not only that, but, "You can control your walk to suit a particular occasion or to send a message. Just as you choose a certain outfit for an important meeting with a client or a silky dress for a special party, you can choose from a variety of walks to find the one that best suits an event." Deborah Perlmutter then described four different walks, "each one suggested for a particular situation or mood. The descriptions tell you how to stand before the first step and then how to move. Follow the directions step by step and then practice to make them natural." The four were The Business Walk, The Sexy Walk, The Athletic Walk, and The Invisible Walk. Instructions for The Sexy Walk began as follows: "Swing your right leg forward from the hip, bending it only slightly at the knee. As you do this, let your hips move naturally. Don't be stiff. Two things should happen. Your left hip should move out and your right hip should move in and twist slightly across the front of your body." Perlmutter then said, "Here's the secret of this walk: Kick a little farther forward than you actually let your foot land. You won't make a great deal of progress, but the effect it creates is worth it."[5]

Wondering whether walking could provide the emotional lift that joggers and swimmers reportedly felt, researcher Sara Snodgrass and colleagues tested the effect of different kinds of walking on the moods of 79 college students. Each student took a three-minute walk in one of three modes: taking long strides, swinging the arms, and fixing their eyes ahead; shuffling along and casting their eyes downward; or with a natural gait.

Shufflers reported greater feelings of depression and fatigue and lower levels of vigor than did the normal walkers and the striders, who showed no difference from each other. Snodgrass said the results suggested that "when we feel down, we can brighten our mood by purposefully walking with vigor." Some earlier research had shown that mimicking the outward signs of a particular mood could, in fact, induce that mood; that caused the researchers to speculate, "If we shuffle along we see ourselves walking as if we felt down, and we decide that we must, therefore, feel down."[6]

In 1987, Robert E. Thayer, a professor of psychology at California State University at Long Beach, compared the effects on perceived energy levels of taking a rapid 10-minute walk to those of eating a candy bar. On 12 different days, 18 college students rated their levels of energy, tension, and fatigue. After taking a walk or eating the candy bar, the subjects rated the three items again at 20 minutes, 60 minutes, and 120 minutes after the activity. Thayer found the students felt much greater energy and less fatigue after the walk than after the snack. That finding held true for all time periods. Although the majority of students felt an increase in energy for at least 20 minutes after snacking, the pick-up was short-lived and showed a marked decrease within two hours. Tensing generally increased after snacking and decreased after a 10-minute walk. Said Thayer, "What is not known by most people is that even a very small amount of exercise can be energizing. And, this type of energy is relatively free of the tension brought on by sugar."[7]

Famed psychologist William James observed back in 1890 that he believed walking alongside a person and observing or copying the walker's gait would reveal what the walker was feeling. German psychologists of the early 1900s argued that a person's character could be ascertained from their style of walking. To test such ideas researchers Joann Montepare, et al., had subjects observe walkers and judge which of the four emotions—happiness, sadness, anger, and pride—were being expressed by the walkers. The walkers read short scenarios that described emotional situations and were told to imagine themselves in that situation and to walk accordingly. For example, the situation for happiness was as follows: "Pretend you are walking down to your friend's room to tell her that you just got a job offer from your first-choice firm." Researchers concluded subjects were able to identify all four emotions from gait information at better than the chance level, although identification of pride was significantly less accurate than were identifications of sadness and anger. Results were also said to reveal that gait characteristics such as the amount of arm swing, stride length, and walking speed differentiated the emotions expressed by the walkers.[8]

Robert Thayer did another study on walking and energy levels, this one in 1988. He had students rate their energy and tension levels and then go for a moderately fast 10-minute walk around the campus. Then they completed the checklist again with the results, as before, indicating people felt less tired and more energetic following the walk. Later he repeated the procedure with subjects who walked on a treadmill in a room with bare walls (to control for attractive campus surroundings, which could have raised energy levels instead of the walk itself). However, again he found the energizing effect held. Cardiologist James Rippe had also found that walking—a three-mile walk in his case—reduced people's anxiety and tension, as well as their blood pressure. Thayer again found the energizing effects lasted for at least an hour; even when measured two hours after the 10-minute walk, the increased energy and reduced tension were still present to a small degree. Thayer concluded, "Walking is, of course, very good physical exercise. Beyond that, it feels good to walk and at moderate walking speeds those good feeling occur right away.... Ten minutes should do it and the benefits—both mental and physical—should last a lot longer."[9]

When researchers D. Jim Walmsley and Gareth J. Lewis observed more than 1,300 pedestrians at 10 different municipalities in Australia and England, they found that walking speed was a function of city size in that pedestrians moved more quickly in big cities than they did in small towns. For example, in Sydney, Australia (population 2,876,508), the walking speed was found to be 1.57 meters per second while in Newcastle (258,972), it was 1.47 and in Armidale (18,722), it was 1.46.[10]

Helen Fisher, an anthropologist at the American Museum of Natural History in New York City, said in 1989 that the way we walk "is a silent flag that reveals the intricacies of our inner lives. Our walk is like a second signature." Dominance and submission, she felt, were the most primitive messages and the most frequent ones projected by the gait. To express status, animals tended to attempt to look larger, walking tall; to express deference most animals made themselves appear small and meek; thus, a self-effacing person hung his head, hunched his shoulders, and cowered as he walked. In a series of studies correlating personality, mood, and gait, psychologist Sara Snodgrass and her students at Skidmore College in Saratoga Springs, New York, explored the language of walking. People were videotaped walking, and then filled out personality profiles. Next, respondents watched the footage and inferred the personalities of the walkers. Among the results were that "The most self-confident, dominant people tended to walk with a long stride and a bounce," while people with a short, mincing step were viewed as subordinate and unsure. Those who swaggered were perceived as lacking self-confidence and sympathy. Foot draggers were thought to be lethargic, and shufflers were perceived as submissive and unorganized. When the judges' ratings were compared with the walkers' personality profiles, noted Fisher, "significant correlations appeared."[11]

In a second test by Snodgrass, a man and a woman were videotaped, each portraying 20 different gaits. Respondents then rated those gaits according to a number of personality characteristics such as self-assured, relaxed, happy, dominant, ambitious, or friendly. Once again, the long stride drew the highest rating while the shuffle was linked with negative traits. The long-striding male was rated more dominant and friendly than was the woman with the long stride and the high-stepping man was rated more relaxed than was the high-stepping woman. On the other hand, the man who walked subserviently was rated lower than the woman who walked in that fashion. Fisher concluded that it seemed more acceptable for a man to "walk tall" and worse for him to "walk small."[12]

Fisher described five common expressive walks: (1) The Choppy Walk — the kind taken by women loaded down with bags — conveyed submissiveness, unfriendliness and frustration; (2) The Duck Walk (exemplified by Charlie Chaplin's Tramp character) — toes pointed out and body swaying a little from side to side — implied an impulsive and independent nature; (3) The Mincing Gait — tiny prim steps that were considered the mark of a victim — which women wearing high heels tended to adopt; (4) The Swagger — with swaying hips leading the way and the upper body leaning back from the pelvis — implied a lack of self-confidence and sympathy; (5) The Depressed Walk, which was the message conveyed by drooping shoulders, a hanging head, and a listless shuffle.[13]

In 1992 *Glamour* magazine presented a rehash of the work by Snodgrass and then commented that if a person wanted to fine-tune the image her gait projected, "it makes sense to consult a pro, but which one?" For image improvement there were said to be many possibilities. "The movement reeducation offered by Laban Movement Analysis or the Alexander Technique can improve the quality of your walk by identifying your habits of misuse and offering constructive substitutes," said Jessica Wolf, certified movement analyst (CMA) in New York City. She recommended about 30 lessons for any kind of change to occur.[14]

Of course there were other explanations for different gaits. Nancy Stedman reported in 1998 that Japanese and U.S. men walked and ran differently because they grew up wearing different kinds of shoes, according to research from Western Michigan University in Kalamazoo. Japanese children traditionally wore flip-flop sandals when learning to walk while Americans wore flexible-soled shoes. As a result, Japanese men tended to plant the entire foot down and leaned forward when they walked; American men struck the ground first with the heel and remained upright.[15]

At the end of 1999 it was reported that a new security system was being developed in Britain that could identify individuals by the unique way in which they walked. One of the developers was Mark Nixon, a computer scientist at the UK's Southampton University. He observed that when people robbed banks they tended to wear motorcycle helmets or some form of disguise, "But you can't disguise your walk without drawing attention to yourself or impeding your escape." Inspired by highly publicized crimes where the suspects were caught on video but with no clear shots of their faces available, Nixon decided to try and find out whether a person's gait could be just as revealing as a snapshot. According to Nixon, his work involving computer analysis of such things as length of a joint, deviation of each joint movement, and so on, was successful, and gait recognition as an identification tool was possible. By using gait recognition, he said, it would be possible to spot a genuinely pregnant woman easily, compared to a female shoplifter who pretended to be in that condition with a bellyful of merchandise. Reportedly, the Southampton project had drawn the interest of UK retailer Marks & Spencer.[16]

Nothing more was heard about the Nixon project but renewed interest in gait recognition was expressed in 2002 with the technology said to be under development at the Georgia Institute of Technology in the U.S., with the aim being to detect, classify, and identify individuals based on the way they walked, and to be able to identify that person up to 500 feet away, day or night, in any weather. Impetus for the renewed interest came from the attacks of September 11, 2001. Georgia Tech research engineer Jon Geisheimer said, "We need technology to find the bad guys at a distance around federal buildings. This is the original application. And after September 11, we began to see the usefulness of those technologies in airports." At the end of 2002, two federally funded studies on gait recognition were underway at Georgia Tech. Early stages of gait recognition technology were expected to serve as a screening tool in conjunction with other biometric methods such as face recognition. Researchers acknowledged that workable gait recognition methods were years in the future.[17]

Rebecca Lee conducted a study in 2001 that examined the association of walking for exercise and mood in sedentary, ethnic minority women (45 percent Latino, 40 percent African-American, seven percent Asian) over a five-month period. Subjects participated in an eight-week program that promoted the adoption of walking for exercise, compared to a control group that remained sedentary. At the start of the study, the subjects reported walking an average of 18.3 minutes a week; by the end of the eight-week study the average was 98.7 minutes per week. Results after eight weeks and at the five-month follow-up revealed the subjects reported significant decreases in depressive mood and increases in vigor compared to the control group. Researchers concluded the increase in walking over the course of the study was associated with changes in vigor and "Limited evidence was found to support a relationship between walking for exercise and mood enhancement in ethnic-minority women."[18]

And just who was it that walked, and how far did they walk?

# 13
# Walking by the Numbers

> "Housewives walk 3,000 miles a year in own homes, survey finds."
>
> New York Times, 1936.

One of the earliest estimates as to distances walked was given by C. N. Holmes in 1919. He said the average distance walked by each person in the United States (man, woman and child) was four miles a day. Thus, the average American walked 120 miles per month, 1,440 miles per year, and 100,000 miles in the Biblical life span of three score and ten.[1]

More figures were presented in 1927 by Dr. Joseph Lelyveld of Boston, Massachusetts, executive director of the National Association for Foot Health. According to him, the average distance walked in a day was almost eight miles. A woman shopper on an average shopping day did about 8.33 miles through the stores; a school girl at school and at play averaged 11.5 miles a day; a boy did 15 miles; a salesgirl averaged eight miles; a steward working in a grill room from 11:00 a.m. to 9:00 p.m. walked 12.5 miles; a letter carrier averaged 22 miles; a department store buyer did seven miles; a golfer playing 18 holes covered 8.5 miles; a female clerical worker in a business office averaged 57 miles a week; and a stenographer covered 43 miles in a week.[2]

Almost a decade later, Lelyveld, then director of research for the National Association of Chiropodists, presented a paper at one of the group's meeting in which he gave the same numbers as in the past. A farmer plowing, he said, averaged 25.5 miles a day, while a housewife walked 3,000 miles a year without ever leaving her house.[3]

That time around, Lelyveld's figures caught the eye of the editor of the *New York Times* who wrote an editorial on the "startling" figures. Summarizing that the farmer at the plow did 25 miles a day, the woman shopper eight miles, the housewife nine miles and the businessman nine to 12 miles during office hours, the editor said "we are a bit doubtful about the figures." He thought the number for the shopper was about right and the plowman's figure "a little hard to accept," but the numbers for the housewife and businessman "simply cannot be visualized."[4]

According to a 1954 account in the *New York Times*, statistics on the oldest form of transportation had been gathered by the Scholl Manufacturing Company of Chicago (maker of foot-related products such as inserts for shoes). Although the article implied the figures were recent and gathered by the Scholl Company, what were presented were the old ones from Lelyveld, including the salesgirl doing eight miles and the female shopper averaging eight miles and a bit.[5]

Figures from the 1970 U. S. census showed almost 300,000 New Yorkers regularly walked to work. While walking to work was holding its own in New York City, it was losing ground nationally to the automobile. According to the United States Bureau of the Census in 1970, 9.5 percent of New York's 3.1 million employed residents walked regularly all the way from their homes to their jobs. It was exactly the same percentage of New Yorkers who in the 1960 census said they walked to work. Nationally, the proportion of Americans who walked to work dropped from 10 percent in 1960 to 7.4 percent in 1970, a decrease from 6.4 million people to 5.7 million. At the same time, the proportion of working Americans who used mass transportation for commuting declined from 12.5 percent to 8.5 percent.[6]

Random interviews with residents in New York and a number of other cities across the nation in 1972 indicated that fear of street crime was increasingly inhibiting them from walking in certain sections of their cites— growing fears being expressed by residents in Boston, New Orleans, Detroit, Chicago, and San Francisco. Also, the number of people who walked to work fluctuated with the thermometer. Of a dozen New Yorkers who were asked about their preference for commuting by foot, virtually all told reporter Robert Lindsey they would not do so after 8:00 p.m. In other cities the percentage of employed residents who regularly walked to work, according to the 1970 census, were; Boston 11.0 percent, New York 9.5 percent, Chicago 8.5 percent, Philadelphia 7.5 percent, and Los Angeles 5.3 percent. Nationally, thought Lindsey, the decline in the number of foot commuters appeared related to the exodus of jobs and many middle-class citizens to the suburbs; the gradual decay of many cities' central business districts; the fear of crime; and the broader availability of the automobile, especially for some people on the lower rungs of the economic ladder.[7]

A 1975 study showed the average pedestrian jaunt in midtown Manhattan was about one-third of a mile. People walked an average of 1,000 feet to lunch, about half as far as they walked to shop. Rain was said to inhibit walking activity by 25 to 50 percent, and weather conditions overall in New York were described as unpleasant for walking approximately 33 percent of the time. Those findings were from a report based on four years of research by the Regional Plan Association. It advocated a new subway station design and the redesign of existing plazas as ways to encourage more walking. One important pedestrian phenomenon it found was the tendency to "platoon"— the bunching up of people because of stop lights and subway train arrivals. Also, about twice as many people were on the sidewalks during peak periods as the average throughout the rest of the day. Because of that, and the design of walkways, pedestrians were reduced to an uncomfortably small amount of space each, which reduced walking speed to half the normal rate.[8]

Princeton University psychologist Dr. Marc H. Bornstein and his anthropologist wife Helen G. Bornstein measured how fast people walked along the main streets of municipalities of varying sizes. In doing so, they confirmed what most people sensed to be true — the bigger the city, the faster its inhabitants walked. They found, for example, that on Flatbush Avenue in Brooklyn people walked at a brisk five feet per second, only a little slower than their counterparts on Wenceslas Square in Prague, who moved at 5.8 feet per second (both cities had populations in excess of one million). By contrast the 365 residents of Psychro, Greece moved at a pace of 2.7 feet per second and the people of Corte, France (population 5,500) went along at 3.3 feet per second. Covering 15 communities in six countries, the study found that a general correlation between population and walking speed existed among municipalities within the individual countries, as well as among municipalities regardless of country. In the three smallest communities people walked at an average pace of 2.7 feet per second, covering 50 feet in 18.4 seconds, while in the three larges cities the average speed was 5.5 feet per second, 50 feet in 9.1 seconds. To conduct the study, the Bornsteins selected the main commercial street of each locality, measured off a 50-foot stretch of sidewalk, and then clocked pedestrians (ones that were alone and unencumbered). The correlation between walking speed and population size was highly significant and unlikely to have been due to chance. As to why such a difference, the Bornsteins speculated that the big cities' streets were full of sights, sounds, noise, and commotion, and walking faster may have made it easier for the pedestrian to keep his attention focused by allowing him to more speedily navigate areas of stimulus overload.[9]

Data from the 1980 census indicated that in metro New York City there were 405,146 people who walked to work —10 percent of all the employed people over the age of 16 who lived in the metro area, an increase over the 9.5 percent from the 1970 census.[10]

Probably nowhere were the numbers of walkers subject to wider fluctuation and lack of standardized definitions than in the number of people who reportedly walked for exercise. In 1982, *Consumers' Research Magazine* said that around half of the 152 million American adults (18 years of age and older) claimed they exercised regularly, and two-thirds of them listed walking as one of their exercise activities. Nearly 35 million Americans said they walked for exercise virtually every day, while another 15 million said they did so two or three times a week. Walking was described as the only exercise in which the rate of participation did not decline in the middle and later years. According to a national survey, the highest percentage of regular walkers (39.4 percent) for any age group was found among males aged 65 and older.[11]

Yet, according to a National Sporting Goods Association survey in 1990, 20.2 million Americans said they walked at least twice a week making that the most popular of 27 categories of sports and fitness activities.[12]

Researchers Paul Siegal, et al., studied the relative contribution of walking to overall leisure-time physical activity, and participation rates among respondents from the 45 states that participated in the 1990 Behavioral Risk Factor Surveillance System (81,557 respondents). They found the percentages of low income, unemployed, and obese persons who engaged in leisure-time physical activity (with a range of 51.1 percent to 57.7 percent for the three subgroups) were substantially lower than the percentage for the total adult population (70.3 percent). In contrast, the prevalence of walking for exercise among those sedentary groups (range of 32.5 percent to 35.9 percent) was similar to that found among the total population (35.6 percent). "Walking appears to be an acceptable, accessible exercise activity, especially among population subgroups with a low prevalence of leisure-time physical activity," concluded the researchers.[13]

Persons who reported walking for exercise in that survey were categorized as either regular walkers (three or more sessions a week of at least 20 minutes per session) or irregular walkers (fewer than three sessions per week and/or less than 20 minutes per session). Of the 81,557 total respondents, 70.3 percent reported having engaged in some physical activity other than their regular job duties during the month before the interview. Rates of participation in such activities decreased with age but increased with income levels. Of the 70.3 percent who reported at least some physical activity, approximately half (35.6 percent of the total sample) were walkers. There was very little variation in walking rates across great income differences. For example, persons with a family income greater than

$50,000 were much more likely to participate in some activity than were those with an income below $10,000 (82.7 percent versus 56.7 percent), but the percentages of people in these groups who walked for exercise were much closer (36.9 percent versus 32.6 percent). Employed persons were more likely to participate in some activity than were those unemployed for a year or more (73 percent versus 51.1 percent), but percentages of people in those groups who walked for exercise were close to equal (33.4 percent versus 32.5 percent). More than half of all the respondents who reported walking for exercise did so on a regular basis. [The exact percentage of regular walkers was not given, but it probably was not a lot greater than half, or it would have been stated — two-thirds for example. Assuming 60 percent would have meant 20 percent of Americans were regular walkers by the definition of three times a week, at least 20 minutes per time. Yet, from the figures above, the data reported in 1982 by *Consumers' Research Magazine* put 35 percent of Americans into the category of those who walked for exercise, 35 million every day and 15 million two or three times a week. Such were the discrepancies in the numbers commonly found in articles.][14]

Of the 50 largest cities in America, the top 10 in terms of percentage of workers aged 16 and older who walked to work (defined as city residents who used walking as their only means of transportation to work in the week preceding the 1990 census) were, based on data from the U.S. Census Bureau for the 1990 census; (1) Boston, 14.0; (2) Pittsburgh, 12.6; (3) Washington, D.C., 11.8; (4) New York, 10.7; (5) Philadelphia, 10.4; (6) San Francisco, 9.8; (7) Buffalo, 8.5; (8) Minneapolis, 7.8; (9) Baltimore, 7.4; (10) Seattle, 7.2.[15]

A national poll of 1,146 adults conducted in 1994 found that more than 40 percent were afraid to walk alone at night within one mile of their home.[16] Journalist John O'Neil reported in 2002 that people in cities and suburbs who lived in homes built before 1974 were almost 50 percent more likely to walk for pleasure than were people whose homes were built after that date. Some 17,000 respondents were asked if they walked a mile or more at least 20 times a month; 11 percent of those living in houses built after 1974 and 16 percent of those in older houses indicated they did. Lead researcher Dr. David Berrigan of the National Cancer Institute explained it was not the house itself but the neighborhood. He concluded that development patterns in the 1950s and 1960s were more conducive to an active lifestyle than development since then.[17]

Also in 2002, a Canadian journalist, Samantha Grice, and her newspaper the *National Post*, did some informal research into the 10,000 step program that had become a minor rage in the U.S. Ten thousand steps was a calorie-burning goal and equivalent to walking about five miles (eight kilometers). As an exercise regimen the idea was to walk 10,000 steps, at least, every day. The *Post* handed out pedometers, asking participants to put one on in the morning as they started their day and to remove it before going to bed. Results were as follows: Graham Rolimieu, freelance illustrator (24 years old, 9,029 steps); Rick Campanelli, MuchMusic disk jockey (age not known, 5,141); David Kines, MuchMusic vice president (40, 5,960); Joann, ER nurse at Toronto General Hospital (51, 11,541); Gio Smaldino, male stylist (32, 3,585); Melissa Pluch, home-based jewelry designer (35, 6,830); Donna Maloney, actor/waitress (26, 10,069); Colleen Mullen, receptionist (57, 4,934); Dr. Edison Barrientos, veterinarian (34, 10,737); Brian Bailey, letter carrier with Canada Post (52, 20,207); Calvin Miller, grade seven student (12, 19,379). None of these people did any extra walking, or running, over the course of the day, except for the student, who did some skipping.[18]

Walking changed dramatically in the 20th century from an activity that was as much intellectual and philosophical as it was an exercise, from an activity that nourished mind and soul as well as body to a purely instrumental activity bound up with numbers and the marketing of incidental paraphernalia. Standards were constantly lowered until the point was reached that someone who walked three times a week for 20 minutes each time was defined as a regular walker, a far cry from earlier times. One of the main reasons for that decline in walking was the automobile and its effects. When the walker came into contact and contest with the automobile he was generally described as a pedestrian. Not everybody was a walker. In fact, most people were not. But everybody was a pedestrian, if only for the time it took to cover a few blocks from a parking lot to an office. The contest between the two was very uneven, as *everything* favored the car.

# 14
# Pedestrians Versus Cars

*"But all this does not alter the incontrovertible fact that many pedestrians are killed and injured because they invade motor vehicle rights of way."*
James Spearing, 1936.

*"Above all, however, the pedestrian is himself to blame.... The experts are agreed that the main reason so many pedestrians are mangled or killed is their own damn foolishness."*
David Wittels, 1949.

*"For one thing, the pedestrian — who is often a hard drinker — is not the type of person who's all that worried about his or her well-being."*
Richard Blomberg, 1993.

*"It is much more acceptable that the victims [pedestrians] are held responsible."*
British Medical Journal, 2002.

Given that a pedestrian weighs next to nothing, compared to a car; given that a pedestrian moves at almost no speed at all, compared to a car; given the impossibility of a pedestrian prevailing or coming out even in a collision with a car, one might have thought some sympathy would be expressed for the pedestrian. However, very little was recorded. Despite the obvious disadvantages faced by the pedestrian, he was mostly portrayed as being at fault, the cause of grief to motorists. According to figures compiled by the Cook County, Illinois, coroner's office in 1923, it was 3.33 times as dangerous to travel on foot in Cook County (in which Chicago is situated) as it was to drive or ride in a car. From December 1, 1922, to November 30, 1923, 539 pedestrians were killed by motor vehicles in Cook County.[1]

When Henry Bliss stepped off a trolley at the corner of Central Park West and 74th Street in New York and was struck and killed by a car driven by Arthur Smith on September 13, 1899, he became, reportedly, America's first recorded pedestrian traffic fatality and ever since that day, wrote William Dean and Simon Breines (in 1975), "a blood bath has been underway."[2] An editorial in the *New York Times* in 1925 declared that something like an "irrepressible conflict" existed between car drivers and pedestrians before it went on in a vague and undefined way to counsel a reasonable approach to the situation from both parties.[3]

Four years later, another editorial in that newspaper noted a suggestion, recently made by a coroner in London, England, that pedestrians injured by cars should be fined for carelessness. Convinced, though, that such a suggestion would never be implemented in America, the editor fumed, "We in America have long since given up the theory that the pedestrian has any rights. He is fair game for the motorist. Whatever the law, in practice he must be a kangaroo. Under no circumstances may he delay a taxi even a fifth of a second."[4]

If the above editor seemed to show at least a little sympathy for the pedestrian, one writing in *The New Statesman* (UK) did not. He hoped the then recently formed Pedestrians' Association would draw up "a scheme for the protection of motorists from suicidal pedestrians. For the suicidal pedestrian is almost as great a trouble on the roads as the murderous [that is, careless] motorist." As far as this article was concerned pedestrians who wandered about in the road and made themselves difficult to pass were practicing "obstruction" and holding up the 20th century. Then the story was related of what had happened in Albania when the authorities resolved that the practice of the residents of Tirana of walking in the middle of the street would cease. Accordingly, soldiers with fixed bayonets had been patrolling the streets for several days and forcing pedestrians to keep to the sidewalks. "If the pedestrians of Tirana had not become a public menace, is it conceivable that they would have been dealt with like a body of insurgents?" concluded the editor.[5]

In 1931 there were 311,910 killed or injured in auto accidents, with 29 percent of those involving pedestrians trying to cross streets at points other than intersections. Next most frequently occurring, in order ranging from 16 percent down to 12 percent, were children playing in the street, pedestrians crossing at uncontrolled intersections, crossing against the light, and stepping from behind parked cars. Connecticut's pedestrian death toll in 1931 was 255, with detailed accounts for 249 of them. One hundred and fifty-eight pedestrians died in traffic accidents at night and 76 during the daytime (15 at dusk). Yet 80 percent of car traffic occurred in the daytime and only 20 percent at night. Therefore, one-fifth of the automobile traffic accounted for over three-fifths of the pedestrian fatalities.[6]

One study found that in Rhode Island in the five-year period 1927–1931, the percentage of traffic accidents due to faults of motorists increased from 66 percent to 90 percent while the percentage due to faults of pedestrians decreased from 30 percent to eight percent. William McAdoo, former police commissioner and later chief city magistrate of New York, expressed his thoughts on the contest between pedestrians and automobiles at an earlier time (before traffic regulations were first adopted in that city in 1903). With regard to that time, McAdoo said, "The jostle and struggle between the driver and pedestrian had been for many, many years a fixed condition, quietly accepted by the multitudes. The driver, on his part, believed that the street belonged exclusively to him and ... he sat on his throne as one beyond the law. The citizens went daily, with more or less courage, through greater perils and dangers than an arctic explorer ... or a hunter of dangerous wild beasts would encounter, glad at times to gain the curb, frequently escaping a violent and cruel death by a hair's breadth."[7]

One decided expression of sympathy for pedestrians came in a 1934 editorial in the *Saturday Evening Post*, which observed that for almost a generation the highway-building program had been gathering speed and momentum. It was a trend that, if anything, had been stimulated by Depression-era public works programs. "Yet it is a curiously stupid fact that the roadways have been constructed, with only insignificant exceptions, without any thought for the pedestrian," complained the editor. That year it was expected 2,000 pedestrians would be killed walking along those highways and 8,000 more injured across America. As to the oft-repeated instruction given to pedestrians to walk facing the traffic in such situations, the *Post* labelled it "deadly," since "Careful studies in several of the most populous states show that injuries to those walking against traffic are more serious than to those walking with it." Concluded the editor, "There is no excuse whatever that so great a system of highways should have been constructed with so inadequate a system of pedestrian paths."[8]

*Chatelaine* magazine published not an article, but 10 small sketches in its February 1937 issue illustrating the 10 most frequent causes of accidents to pedestrians in Canada. Each showed the pedestrian at fault; for example, "Crossing without proper care at intersections without lights" and "Waiting for, or getting on or off street cars without proper care." The tone of the piece was that pedestrians were always to blame for traffic accidents to which they were a party.[9]

Another who blamed the pedestrian was James Spearing, who wrote a column about automobiles that ran regularly in the *New York Times*. In his May 24, 1936, column he announced he was back "to introduce additional evidence in the case against the pedestrian." He briefly noted there were some bad motorists but moved quickly to his main point: "But all this does not alter the incontrovertible fact that many pedestrians are killed and injured because they invade motor vehicle rights of way." As evidence, he cited the accident report for New York City for April 1936, in which 397 accidents were reported that involved pedestrians trying to cross streets. Of that number, 133 involved people not using designated crossings, and 172 involved people crossing against lights. Thus, concluded Spearman, there were 305 out of 397 accidents "in which the pedestrians were definitely in the wrong, no matter how careless the motorists may have been." To make matters worse, moaned the columnist, "a more sensitive driver may suffer serious nervous disorders if his car kills or injures a pedestrian even though the accident was not his fault."[10]

A clinic for testing and instructing pedestrians, established in Wichita, Kansas, in 1938, was set up on the assumption, said a news account, that "Pedestrians, in a great many cases, know nothing whatever about cars." Reportedly, those walkers were completely unaware of the difficulty of quickly stopping, had never tried to see through a clouded windshield, were clueless about skidding on icy roads, and so on. Among their almost limitless faults, pedestrians were unable to judge the speed of an approaching car. Therefore, in the Wichita clinic, for example, miniature cars operated at various speeds controlled by the instructor served as a means to teach students that essential type of judgment.[11]

Going a little further along the same lines was a 1939 editorial in *Scientific American*. After noting that 15,000 pedestrians were killed yearly in traffic accidents and that the majority of those victims did not know how to drive, the editor went on to suggest that everybody, regardless of age, should learn how to drive, even those who did not intend to ever do so or did not own or have access to a car. "If these pedestrians will take the time and trouble to learn how to drive a motor car, even though they may never have occasion to do so, they will have laid a foundation of knowledge that will be as important to their futures as the simple rules of health and sanitation."[12]

Reporter David Wittels titled an article about pedestrians versus cars that appeared in the *Saturday Evening Post* in January 1949, "They Ask to Be Killed." As a subhead, he used the following: "Do you invite massacre by your own carelessness? Here's how thousands have committed suicide by scorning laws that were passed to keep them alive." He called the situation between pedestrians and motorists "a feud.... In this feud the pedestrian practically always loses.... He literally would be safer on a lion-infested African veldt or in man-eating tiger territory than he is crossing a downtown street at dusk." According to Wittel's numbers the pedestrian "is being slaughtered at the rate of about thirty a day and mangled at the rate of nearly 700 a day." In the previous 10 years, cars were said to have killed close to 113,000 pedestrians, and more than 6,000 bicyclists.[13]

Wittels, in a brief mention, gave some of the blame to drivers and some to state and municipal authorities as most traffic laws "are primarily for the benefit of motorists and to expedite vehicular traffic." But he saved most of his attack for the walkers: "Above all, however, the pedestrian is himself to blame. In this bloody feud he is his own worst enemy. The experts are agreed that the main reason so many pedestrians are mangled or killed is their own damn foolishness. And as one possible cure, some of the experts argue that foolish and reckless pedestrians should be put in jail." Then Wittels cited a survey by the National Safety Council that purportedly indicated that two out of every three pedestrians killed by motor vehicles "were either violating a traffic law or acting in an obviously unsafe manner." A study done in Cleveland reportedly concluded that 90 percent of the walkers killed and 65 percent of those injured "were either drunk, crossing against the lights or jaywalking."[14]

An unsigned article in *Harper's Magazine* in 1957 described pedestrians as a "persecuted majority." Cited was a safety booklet put out by the Travelers Insurance company that had a section called "Actions of pedestrians resulting in deaths and injuries," which the writer felt might more accurately have been called "Actions of motorists resulting in the massacre of helpless pedestrians." As an example, he cited the fact that 17,730 pedestrians were injured in 1954 crossing the street with a green light, while almost the same number (18,500) were injured crossing against the light. In his view, this meant it made almost no difference what the pedestrian did. Nearly 11,000 pedestrians were injured (and 340 killed), he reported, "not on roadway," which conjured up images for him of cars pursuing them everywhere. Also, motorists killed 280 men working on the roads and injured 6,370 more. This observer felt that to motorists, pedestrians were "the enemy" and that all the rules and regulations were made to favor the motorist over the pedestrian. Someone once wrote, "A pedestrian is a man in danger of his life; a walker is a man in possession of his soul," and for the *Harper's* reporter the first part of that observation was still true but the second part had become dated.[15]

The French architect Le Corbusier said in 1932 that it was necessary to make a definite distinction between the pedestrian and the vehicle, "which should never be allowed to meet." His solution was to put both buildings and motor roads on stilts, leaving to the walker "the surface of the city, all the surface, the earth." He wanted to see the pedestrian put on the ground with a network of avenues at his disposal that ran in all directions in the midst of parks and lawns. Writing in 1957, journalist Lois Balcom agreed with the idea of separating cars and people but said that nothing had happened along those lines and all the changes and regulations such as parking lots, street widening, traffic light timing cycles, and so on, had been done to maximize vehicle speeds and convenience while leaving the pedestrian to his own devices. Balcom told the story of a man in New York's Westchester County who had recently been arrested for walking to work. On his way to the restaurant where he worked, he got off a bus on the far side of the New York State Thruway and walked across its several lanes (an offense) to get to the restaurant. The restaurant had been marooned on an island between the newly completed thruway and an existing parkway and was left with literally no legal access to its site except by private car.[16]

Britain's respected business magazine, *The Economist*, came out with its own anti-pedestrian article in 1972, wherein it said, "Although Britain is about the safest country to be in a car, it is murderous for pedestrians, and the mothers of Britain share the blame." That was because a report by the Road Research Laboratory indicated 33 percent to 50 percent of three- to eight-year-olds (depending on age) included the street among their usual play places. Pedestrian casualties per 1,000 population were said to be worse in Britain than in the U.S. or any other European country. Apart from the very old, children were the most frequent victims and nearly 12,000 under the age of 15 were killed or seriously injured each year. Speaking about pedestrians of all ages, *The Economist* went on to say, "Britain is a long way behind other countries in being stern with pedestrians. In fear of the police, Americans and Japanese wait obediently by the pedestrian lights until told they can go.... Concern about pedestrian behaviour is getting so great that there is a growing movement to make pedestrians subject to statutory control." However, such control was difficult to achieve in Britain because the British did not carry identity cards. An experiment in trying to penalize pedestrians in London a few years earlier led to an "extraordinary number" of the accused giving their names as John Smith.[17]

Susan Baker, with the Department of Public Health Administration, Johns Hopkins University School of Hygiene and Public Health, gave a presentation in 1973 at the annual meeting of the American Public Health Association. She started off by asking the question, "How can you kill ten thousand Americans a year without public outrage?" Her answer was, "Run them down with a hundred million cars." Baker observed that each year Americans traveled more miles in their cars, and each year they walked less. Yet in the previous decade, the per capita pedestrian death rate had increased by 20 percent.[18]

Baker then compared pedestrian traffic deaths in Baltimore, Maryland, and in Rio de Janeiro, Brazil, for 1970. For Baltimore, if the age distribution of victims was graphed it looked like the letter V, with the bottom at age 30. Twenty-five percent of the victims were children under 10; 25 percent were aged 65 or older; 25 percent were under the influence of alcohol. It meant that 75 percent of all the pedestrians killed in Baltimore were very young, elderly, or intoxicated — "the kinds of people least likely to perceive adequately and respond appropriately to the signals and hazards of the traffic environment," she said. For Rio, the graph was shaped like a pyramid with the peak at age 40, and relatively few young children and elderly people and not many under the influence of alcohol. Overall, only 25 percent of the Rio victims were either less than 10, 65 plus, or under the influence of alcohol. Most were sober, working-age adults. For sober adults in the 15 to 64 age group, the per capita death rate in Rio was 20 times the Baltimore rate. "But a substantial proportion of apparently able-bodied people among pedestrian fatalities should serve as a flag, calling attention to a difficult task that involves unusual environmental hazards," Baker added. An extreme example in Rio was a superhighway that split a densely populated community. A 15-mile stretch of it claimed 200 pedestrian deaths in 1970, out of a total of 1,000. There were pedestrian bridges along the way over the highway but they were infrequently placed and involved climbing stairs so many people chose to take a chance on crossing the busy six-lane highway.[19]

Baker argued that the transportation system should be designed around the pedestrian, not the car; that America should move away from "the principle that moving people in cars quickly is more desirable than moving people on foot safely" and that it was time to shift the burden away from the pedestrian — who paid with his time, energy, and even his life — and onto the vehicle. "In any encounter with a moving vehicle, the pedestrian will lose," she said; "Is it fair that he must function in a system designed by and for motorists." She concluded, "But until planners everywhere represent the interests of the pedestrian, rather than the interests of those with a much larger economic stake in the system, we can expect little change in the grim statistics on pedestrians."[20]

*Changing Times* magazine ran a 1979 article in which it complained that "Erring pedestrians gamble with their lives every day as they dash, dart, jaywalk and daydream across highways and byways." Listed were some of the foolish things pedestrians did and the mistakes they made such as "Failing to get a driver's attention." Noted was the fact most states had laws protecting pedestrians — such as cars having to yield at crosswalks having no signal — but the piece admitted, "often drivers don't honor this and police give low priority to enforcement." Nowhere in the article was mention made that the driver was the one at fault.[21]

William Whyte delivered a talk in New York City in 1982 called "Pedestrian Life: Tokyo and New York." He found that the same amount and kind of pedestrian congestion existed in Tokyo as in New York and that the people in both cities were skilful pedestrians, which was remarkable "since both cities are equally hostile to pedestrians." For example, in New York, he said any time a decision had to be made favoring either cars or pedestrians, "cars always win."[22]

Whyte had documented street life in America for many years. At a talk he gave in Colorado in 1984 at the Third Annual Pedestrian Conference, he said that one of the highest aims of modern planning was the separation of vehicular and pedestrian traffic. Supposedly, he argued, it was all done for the good of the pedestrian — but not really, because separation was even better for cars since they could travel faster and did not have to stop to let a bunch of pedestrians cross. As an example, he cited pedestrian bridges that pedestrians often "sensibly" avoided since they involved extra time and effort to use — going out of one's way, climbing stairs, and the like. But, argued Whyte, it was in the division of space that the pedestrian got the shortest shrift, because in almost all American cities the bulk of the space was given over to roadways for vehicles, the least to sidewalks for pedestrians. In many areas, of course, the sidewalks were not crowded, but that was usually the result of a dead downtown area. When a city had a vibrant central business district, continued Whyte, "the space imbalance can have severe effects. Not only are the sidewalks heavily crowded at peak time; there is a lack of space for such simple amenities as a place to sit." On New York's Lexington Avenue (between 57th and 58th Streets) the road was 50 feet wide and the sidewalk 12.5 feet wide. Each day, 22,000 people used the sidewalks on the east side and 19,000 on the west side, for a total of 41,000, with an effective sidewalk width of less than 12 feet given such things as trash cans, mailboxes, fire hydrants, and poles that lined part of the sidewalk. During the same period, 25,000 people traversed the block in vehicles. Yet the space allocation was about two-to-one in favor of vehicles, Whyte thought it should be reversed.[23]

Daniel Ross's article was supposed to be partly humorous but any humor it may have contained failed to mask the underlying hatred and loathing of pedestrians. It was one of the most vitriolic of the anti-pedestrian pieces and was published in 1987 in a perhaps appropriate forum — *Motor Trend* magazine. In his view, of course, everything was the fault of the pedestrian. "But how many times have you had to screech to an abrupt halt, risking a rear-end collision, as some wank strides confidently into the middle of traffic without even a common-sense look over the shoulder?" he grumbled. After a brief mention of the pedestrian right-of-way laws and conceding that such rules should exist, he added, "but it fails to take into account the sort of baffling disregard for personal safety most foot traffic exhibits." Continuing his diatribe, Ross fumed, "The law of averages insists that somewhere in a life peppered with near misses is a Buick with a stupid pedestrian's name on it. The jerk, however, the walking goofbucket, believes that deadly Buick has some other goofbucket's name on it." Concluding his rant, he offered the following: "All kidding aside, pedestrians must begin to watch out for themselves. The quality of walking stupidity observable from behind a car steering wheel is astonishing, and it definitely isn't funny ... you folks on foot just are not holding up your end."[24]

Although pedestrian traffic deaths edged downward in the early 1990s, more than five pedestrians were killed by vehicles in an average week in New York City. There were 277 pedestrian deaths in New York in 1992, compared to 296 in 1991 and 366 in 1990. Nationally, there were about 97,000 pedestrian accidents in 1992, 67,000 of which were categorized by the authorities as minor to moderate, 24,450 as severe, and 5,546 as fatal. That was the lowest number of fatalities nationwide since 1927 when pedestrian fatality statistics were first reported. Peak times for pedestrian deaths were between 7:00 p.m. and 9:00 p.m. in New York, with the second and third most likely times being at noon and at 5:00 p.m. Although, nationally, Friday and Saturday nights were the most dangerous times for pedestrians, in New York City the riskiest time to take a walk was Wednesday at noon. Half of all pedestrian fatalities took place while the person was crossing the street. Sixty percent of all deaths of pedestrians aged 16 and older who were killed at night in 1991 involved victims with a blood alcohol concentration of 0.10 or higher — a level sufficient to have a driver arrested for impaired driving. In New York City in 1992, 37 percent of the walkers killed showed traces of alcohol and/or other drugs. People aged 65 and over accounted for 33 percent of all the pedestrian deaths in New York although they made up only 13 percent of the city's population. Nearly one in three traffic deaths in Great Britain involved a pedestrian; in the U.S. it was one in seven. Males made up 62 percent of the pedestrian deaths in Manhattan while nationally the male death rate was twice that for women. There were even worse places. In New Delhi, India, four times as many people died in traffic accidents as were murdered. During a single year in the early 1980s, over 26,000 people died on Indian roads; that was about half the total traffic deaths in America, although the U.S. had nearly 40 times as many motor vehicles.[25]

According to Richard Blomberg, president of Dunlap & Associates—a "human factors" research company that was said to have undertaken significant studies of traffic safety issues— 30 percent to 50 percent of all pedestrian deaths in traffic incidents for people over 14 years of age involved walkers with significant amounts of alcohol in the blood. He thought this "problem" was usually not mentioned in media accounts and that some police departments did not think to check for that link. Because of that, a knowledge gap existed and, for example, bartenders—well aware of the drinking/driving link—sometimes suggested drunk patrons walk home. Those drunk walkers caused many problems, with Blomberg citing the highly improbable one of a driver being injured after he struck a drunk pedestrian: What if the walker flew up and went through the windshield? Other negative side effects cited from drunk walkers included increased insurance rates and lost productivity and mental anguish in the driver. It was all, of course, little more than an attempt to find another way to blame the victim. "This is an extremely difficult problem," said Blomberg; "For one thing, the pedestrian—who is often a hard drinker—is not the type of person who's all that worried about his or her well-being."[26]

Journalist Jay Walljasper observed in 1994 that one-sixth of those who died in traffic accidents were pedestrians, with the streets being doubly dangerous for the disabled, the elderly, and children. Michael Replogle, a transportation policy analyst at the Environmental Defense Fund, commented, "We are in danger of losing a basic human right, the right to walk in your own neighbourhood." Australian transportation analyst David Engwicht noted that, instead of wandering and playing in the streets, children had to be kept indoors when they were not supervised. Instead of being outside playing, they watch *Sesame Street*, a fictional street where children played safely and went exploring. As Engwicht pointed out, for 10,000 years city streets had been places to socialize and play, as well as serving as pathways for all forms of transportation—carriages, wagons, pack animals, and most of all, people. But now, streets were reserved for the exclusive use of automobiles. Although that shift started in the U.S. it became the rule across most of the world, even in developing countries where only a very small percentage of the population owned cars. A 1988 Pacific News Service account described street life in Bangkok, Thailand: "Crossing a thoroughfare is generally a life-threatening undertaking.... For the most part pedestrians stand on street corners, with intense and strained faces, gauging the traffic and darting between lanes when the flow temporarily wanes."[27]

Walljasper argued that in their campaign to claim sole ownership of the streets, drivers were helped by several generations of transportation planners "who single-mindedly focus on promoting the smooth and speedy flow of vehicles. Pedestrians and bicyclists rarely figure in their plans, except as nuisances who slow down traffic." That emphasis on speed made it more dangerous for the walkers. A study by the UK government showed that at 20 miles per hour, only five percent of vehicle/pedestrian collisions resulted in deaths to the walker, but at 40 miles per hour, 85 percent claimed a pedestrian life. "Modern urban design — vast parking lots, busy driveways, buildings set way back from the street, and sidewalks unprotected from rushing traffic — adds to this process by making the person on foot feel like an alien from another planet," he added. When people felt it was not safe to walk, they drove more, thought Walljasper, and drove more of their children to school and other activities and thus set up a vicious cycle by creating more traffic.[28]

In his 1994 article on the car/pedestrian situation, journalist Robert Yeager began by noting that every year in the U.S. more than 90,000 pedestrians were struck by vehicles and nearly 5,500 of them were killed. Overall, pedestrians accounted for up to 50 percent of all traffic fatalities in large cities. Federal estimates put the nation's annual medical costs and lost-employment costs of pedestrian/vehicle crashes at $8.5 billion. The Insurance Institute for Highway Safety (IIHS) in Arlington, Virginia, reviewed all fatal pedestrian crashes in the U.S. between 1991 and 1993 that involved single vehicles and that at least partly resulted from the drivers' failure to obey a traffic signal or sign. In about half of those collisions, the drivers were not charged with any violations. Electronic cameras photographed over 250,000 automobile red-light runners in less than two years at 18 New York intersections (about 130 per intersection per week). As to why there were so many violations of that law and others, E. Scott Geller, psychology professor at Virginia Polytechnic Institute and State University in Blacksburg, remarked, "There are no negative consequences of their behaviour. We even get rewarded for disobeying the laws—we get to our destination faster." John C. Gleeson, police captain at San Francisco's traffic division, saw "a real change in driver attitudes toward pedestrians. There's no civility, no respect. Drivers seem to think 'If I can save two seconds and run you over, I'll do it.'"[29]

For Yeager, one of the most alarming aspects of the situation was that "drivers who hit pedestrians often go unpunished. Many are never arrested; those who are taken into custody usually get just a small fine or a temporary license suspension." Said John Moffat, the director of Washington State's Traffic Safety Commission, "Drivers in these accidents typically say they 'didn't see' the pedestrian, and invariably they're forgiven." Other IIHS statistics revealed that nearly 20 percent of the motorists who killed pedestrians simply drove away. "In most states the vehicle code places no effective sanctions on drivers who hit and kill those on foot," observed Bill Wilkinson, the executive director of the Washington, D.C.-based Pedestrian Federation of America. "It's hard to prove that a bad driver is guilty of felony charges such as vehicular manslaughter or vehicular homicide. Prosecutors must show that the driver drove in a reckless fashion, with no regard for the safety of others." Yeager added that making matters worse was the fact the streets were designed to put walkers at a disadvantage by such things as right turns on a red light and short walk cycles on traffic lights. Jeffrey Zupan, senior transportation fellow at New York's Regional Plan Association, said that even at the best of times "pedestrians get the short end of the stick. The whole philosophy of traffic engineers is to maximize the speed of vehicular traffic." For too long, declared Moffat, "pedestrians have been treated as a hindrance. We must demand that they be treated as part of the traffic flow. Americans have become accustomed to pedestrian deaths—and that's got to stop."[30]

Between 1986 and 1995 an average of 6,129 pedestrians were struck and killed by vehicles each year on America's streets and highways, according to National Highway Traffic Safety Administration data. Also, an estimated 110,000 pedestrians were injured annually, with the elderly most at risk.[31] In 1993, traffic accidents killed more than 40,000 people in North America, with a further 2.3 million injured. After 1983, said journalist Alan Durning, the amount of driving increased even faster than the number of automobiles. The average vehicle in the states of Idaho, Oregon, and Washington covered 11 miles per person per day in 1957; by 1993 that figure stood at 25 miles. People were driving longer distances, but most of the increase was due to people getting in their cars more often. They were driving on 90 percent of the trips they took, a figure that had been rising for decades at the expense of trains, buses, bicycles, and walking. One reason for that change was sprawl. The percentage of people who lived in suburbs in Idaho, Oregon and Washington rose from seven percent in 1950 to 30 percent in 1990—a change that reflected national trends. It was a mass migration made possible by the automobile; in turn, it had made the car indispensable. People who lived in typical households in the suburbs of those northwestern states owned one car per driver and got in their cars 10 times a day.[32]

According to a 1998 report from the Washington, D.C.-based Surface Transportation Policy Project (STPP), Americans below the age of 19 faced a far greater risk of death from walking than from any more attention-getting causes such as E. coli outbreaks, accidental shootings, and airbag deployments. For example, in 1996, 837 young pedestrians were killed by cars; only 23 were killed by airbags. That same year, over 4,300 adult pedestrians were killed, with walkers regularly accounting for around 12 percent of all traffic-related deaths and serious injuries. By taking serious or fatal pedestrian accidents per 100,000 people and adjusting that to the percentage of the population who walked to work, the STPP devised a "pedestrian danger index." Phoenix got a high 63, New York a safer 28. At the top of the list of most dangerous cities for walkers was Orlando, Florida, with a score of 95, while at the bottom, with a 16, was the Cincinnati/Hamilton region of Ohio. STPP president Roy Kleinitz blamed much of the situation on transportation policies that always favored the motorist and the ever-increasing urban sprawl. All of that contributed to less and less walking and that, in turn, contributed to a growing problem with obesity in America. Said Kleinitz, "Where walking is safe and convenient, more people walk.... We need to stop building communities that treat walkers like the enemy."[33]

As the 1990s progressed, fewer pedestrians were being killed or injured by cars in America — over 5,000 killed and about 77,000 injured in 1997, according to a report from the Insurance Institute for Highway Safety. The situation was worse in big cities, where more than a third of those killed in motor vehicle accidents were walkers. Pedestrian deaths may have been down because Americans were walking less and driving more, but the report admitted the cause of the decline was hard to pinpoint. Between 1975 and 1997, pedestrian deaths dropped by 29 percent. Children aged five to 15 had the highest injury rates; adults aged 65 and over were less likely to get hit by a car but they were more likely to die from a collision. In the U.S., pedestrians accounted for 13 percent of all motor vehicle deaths; in Russia it was 40 percent; 38 percent in Poland; 36 percent in Israel; and over 50 percent in Ethiopia.[34]

Over the course of 1999 (the year of the Columbine school massacre), 28 students nationwide were killed in schools, while 840 young people under the age of 20 were killed while struck by cars as they walked. Yet, said reporter Gregg Easterbrook, such pedestrian deaths drew no notice and no action. He wondered if perhaps we heard so little about pedestrian deaths (around 5,000 in total, yearly) because many of the victims were poor or immigrants. In Fairfax County, Virginia (a suburb of Washington, D.C.) 23 percent of the walkers killed between 1993 and 1998 were Hispanics although they were just eight percent of the county's population. Reportedly, studies in California and other states had also shown that pedestrian deaths occurred disproportionately among Hispanics and the poor. "Another reason we ignore these deaths is that it is easy to blame the victim," said Easterbrook, such as by inferring they were wearing the wrong color of clothing, or they had no business trying to cross such a busy street away from an intersection, and so forth. "But pedestrian deaths aren't mostly the fault of pedestrians; they're mostly the fault of drivers," he stated. Measured by collision deaths per mile traveled, it was 36 times more dangerous to walk than to be in a car, according to the Surface Transportation Policy Project.[35]

Nor was the antipedestrian stance exclusive to America. Writing in 2001 in the *British Medical Journal*, Zosia Kmietowicz cited a report published by a cross-party committee of UK members of Parliament, which declared, "For more than 50 years Britain's government and city planners have sidelined the rights of pedestrians in favour of cars, turning walking into an 'even more unpleasant' experience." Despite the advantages of walking, people in the UK were doing it less, said the report from the House of Commons select committee on the environment, transport, and regional affairs. According to the report the government had promoted car travel because it was "terrified of appearing anti-car." Between the mid 1980s and the late 1990s the number of trips made on foot fell by 20 percent, and it was predicted the trend would continue "unless action was taken to encourage walking." Concluded the committee, "Pedestrians have been treated with contempt. In a myriad of ways when we walk we are treated with less respect than when we drive. We are carolled behind long lengths of guard railing, forced into dark and dangerous subways and made to endure long waits at pedestrian crossings."[36]

Much of the *British Medical Journal's* May 11, 2002, issue was devoted to what it editorially called "the war on the world's roads." It was a special issue on pedestrians versus the automobile. In the words of the editor, "War is often waged by the powerful on the weak. In this case, the interests of pedestrians, cyclists and other vulnerable road users are pitted against the powers that stand to profit from increasing global motorisation." Every day, it was said, about 3,000 people died and 30,000 people were seriously injured on the world's roads. Noted in those figures was a class distinction, in that low-income people and children were disproportionately the victims of such collisions, both in rich countries and in poor nations. "As in other wars, propaganda is an important weapon. It is not in the interests of those who sell road transport to allow the private trouble of road death and injury to become a public issue," stated the editor; "The idea that governments and the motor manufacturing industry have a major responsibility is not for public consumption. It is much more acceptable that the victims are held responsible."[37]

Ever since the car arrived en masse early in the 20th century and the war on the roads got underway, efforts have been made, and are still being made, to control or regulate the pedestrians. Some of those efforts presented themselves as being for the benefit mainly of the pedestrian, but at the back of all such measures and attempts has been a regulation actually for the benefit of motorists. Any benefit to pedestrians was never more than secondary. In more recent times the regulation of pedestrians has taken on a somewhat more scientific cast, as the walker was often studied in conjunction with control and regulation.

# 15

# Regulating Pedestrians, to 1950

*"180-second intervals [at traffic lights] make it almost impossible to control pedestrians."*
                                              E. B. Lefferts, 1927.

*"Clearly most jay-walker laws for pedestrian control discriminate unfairly in favor of the motorist."*
                                              Myron Stearns, 1930.

*"Legislation has been aimed almost entirely at the motorist and the pedestrian has been permitted to be as careless and unreasonable as he pleases."*
                    J. W. Frazer, Chrysler vice president, 1936.

*"We are accustomed to move freely and naturally and would resent a police regulation which might catch the pedestrian unaware when he cannot realize the necessity of such interference."*
                    New York City Mayor Fiorello La Guardia, 1936.

In all cities one of the major banes to planners, police departments, traffic directors, and so on, has been, and remains, the dreaded jaywalker [crossing the street where there was no intersection, as in the middle of the block, or crossing at an intersection controlled by stop lights but crossing against the lights]. A 1926 editorial in the trade journal *Engineering News-Record* fumed that such behavior had to be regulated and stopped: "In arriving at the conclusions that pedestrians as well as vehicular traffic must be controlled the Chicago investigators have come to the attitude of mind to which the directors of traffic in every large city must certainly come." As to why more cities had not already moved to regulate such behavior, the editor thought planners in many cities were afraid to try to change the habits of the 60 percent of the people of a city who, he thought, practiced jaywalking. But, urging more cities to action the editor remarked that many cities had regulated the behavior and were then reaping the benefits [left unstated] of the effort. Taking a hard line, the piece thundered, "Absolute prohibition of pedestrian violation of crossing signals is necessary, with immediate arrest of violators." Experience was said to have shown that in cities such as Los Angeles, after a preliminary few weeks of resentment of the new regulations, the pedestrian himself "sees the benefit of control and thereafter operation becomes as automatic as it is for motors." Such reform in cities across America was mandatory, declared the editor, "if we are to continue to use our streets."[1]

An ordinance that went into effect in New York City on January 1, 1927, gave walkers the right-of-way over cars at intersections "where no police officer is present and no traffic control system is in operation." Drivers were required to slow or stop in order to permit pedestrians to cross. Commenting on that ordinance, the *New York Times* remarked that, up to then, "Everything has been done to expedite motor traffic — quite correctly — but the poor pedestrian has been left to save his own skin — or break his neck, as the case may be — when it comes to getting across the streets."[2]

Oakland, California, set up its system of traffic control signals in 1927 after city engineers had visited other cities to study those systems. On those visits they found that "Everywhere they were confronted with elaborate automatic devices for vehicular control, but the pedestrian was seemingly ignored." With regard to the three-light system (today's now-standard-everywhere red, yellow, and green), Oakland engineers felt the yellow light only served as a signal to motorists to beat the red light, and that situation further endangered the pedestrian. At the time, traffic control signals were in use in a great many cities but the visiting engineers found little uniformity, with types ranging from semaphores to light signals to audible signals, or to some combination of types. Selected by Oakland was a three-light (red and green used in the usual way) signal with a vibrating bell, hung at all four corners of an intersection. With the red light on, the yellow light (marked "ped'n" for pedestrian) flashed and gave walkers a four- to seven-second start on vehicles. After that interval, the red and yellow lights both went off and the green light came on.[3]

Later in 1927, Los Angeles adopted its own traffic control signal system, selecting the same one as Oakland (that is, an advance yellow for walkers). E. B. Lefferts, with the public safety department of the Automobile Club of Southern California at Los Angeles, explained that when his city instituted its pedestrian regulation it used a public relations campaign to make it acceptable. Every radio station in the city broadcast the same information regarding the new ordinance at 8:00 p.m. each night during the week before the ordinance went into effect. Over a quarter of a million copies of summaries of the ordinance were printed and distributed to the public. [Such traffic control systems were installed in a time period when most people did not own cars, with the ordinances often regarded more as pedestrian control systems than motor vehicle control, the benefit accruing to the rapidly swelling population of vehicles]. Of the 371 mechanical stoplights introduced into Los Angeles, 81 were located in the downtown area and those 81 were controlled by 16 different timing cycles. The yellow advance pedestrian light varied from six to nine seconds in length while the green "Go" light for vehicles was never longer than 36 seconds, making the complete cycle range from 68 to 90 seconds. According to Lefferts, in some cities the Go light had been set as long as 180 seconds, and "180-second intervals make it almost impossible to control pedestrians." He added, "The pedestrian does not resent being regulated when he realizes that he is getting a fifty-fifty break with the motorist, which is the case if he is not required to wait an unreasonable length of time on the corner...." At Los Angeles intersections controlled by police officers when the new system took effect, arrests of violating walkers were not usually made. Normally, the policeman blew his whistle and ordered the person back to the curb, or physically took his arm and escorted him back. Either way, this was defined as "ridicule" and felt to be more effective in changing behavior than other measures.[4]

At the 1927 annual convention of the National Highway Traffic Association, a report submitted by its Committee on Pedestrian Traffic — Regulation and Enforcement argued that if pedestrian regulations were simply added to existing law they would not be effective — a public relations campaign would be necessary. "Better pedestrian conduct is going to depend almost entirely upon the magnitude and the effectiveness of the educational measures instituted," said the report. With respect to the protection of pedestrians at uncontrolled intersections (no mechanical system, no police officers) the committee had nothing to say except it "has been unable to agree upon a recommendation." At controlled intersections (either mechanically or officer controlled), it recommended pedestrians have the right-of-way over turning vehicles and "an interval should be provided during which no vehicular traffic should enter the intersection.... This interval should be of sufficient length to allow for a complete pedestrian crossing." [While the advance light for walkers— with no car movement during that interval— was not uncommon during the early years of traffic control signal systems it vanished fairly quickly. Illustrating the dominance of vehicles was the fact that if any advance cycle was built into the traffic control systems in modern times it was only an advance green for left-turning vehicles at busy intersection.] Concluded the report, "Pedestrian control should be attempted only after a thorough and adequate campaign of public education."[5]

City planner J. Haslett Bell wrote in 1927 that, within the previous 12 years, city planning had made great strides but now the pedestrian had to be considered more in city planning, which to then had catered to the automobile. One thing he urged was, "Jay walking must be eliminated in the congested districts. Jay walking is one of the greatest causes of street accidents. It has been found that the rigid enforcement of regulations prohibiting jay walking has greatly increased the capacity of both the roadway and the sidewalk." However, lamented Bell, "There is no traffic more difficult to control than pedestrians, but by rigid and constant measures proper walking habits can be given to the public." He wanted to see an end to the hindering of pedestrian traffic on sidewalks by businesses that put out signs, tables, shrubs, and so forth, on the walkways. Other items to consider, commented Bell, were overhead pedestrian street crossings and subways as a means to carry pedestrians under busy streets.[6]

Foster Ware wrote an article about the problems of being a pedestrian in New York City, even though that individual was a "free man" and not regulated like cars. Ware described him as a free man because in New York at uncontrolled intersections the pedestrian had the right of way and jaywalking was not them barred in the city. Still, with all those rights, the pedestrian was aware of the "futility of attempting to exercise these rights." Concluded Ware, "Law or no law, he no longer is a free agent. No one knows it better than the pedestrian himself. The hunted and often terror-stricken look he wears testifies eloquently to the kind of existence he is leading." As far as Ware was concerned, "A successful pedestrian today must be spry, must be alert, must be a good picker of openings and, above all, must defer to the motorist whenever it comes to a showdown."[7]

Around 1929, the U.S. District Court of Appeals declared that the pedestrian who started to go across the street while a green light was on had the right-of-way until he reached the other curb — even though the light changed to red before he reached the other sidewalk. Reporter Lewis Nichols was another who believed that, regardless of what the laws said or what the courts decided, pedestrians were advised to go slowly in claiming their rights, especially since "The police are not rabid partisans of the pedestrian."[8]

One of Ware's New York City walker freedoms disappeared on May 19, 1930, when that city's pedestrians came under police control as regulations against jaywalking went into effect at 8:00 a.m. with police officers ready to give summonses to walkers who disregarded traffic signals. Under the regulations, pedestrians were not allowed to cross a roadway anywhere except at an intersection or at a marked crosswalk. At uncontrolled crossings, the pedestrian had the right-of-way. At controlled intersections, the walker could cross only with the light or on the direction of a police officer. According to the account, there had been other attempts to curb jaywalking in New York but none of them had been as serious as this effort. Joseph Beihilf, counsel for the Park Avenue Association, complained, "It can scarcely be said a pedestrian's jaywalking is dangerous to an automobile or its occupants."[9]

On May 19, the New York City Police Department assigned 25 patrolmen to four different intersections to start the campaign and to be on the lookout for violators of the new jaywalking rules. And there was no shortage of them. To some of the jaywalkers the patrolmen gave "advice and instruction," but to 16 of the more "flagrant" offenders they gave summonses. Also, the police issued summonses to 22 motorists for violations involving pedestrians. Most common among those was a motorist tactic still much used today—turning right on green but trying to anticipate the exact moment the light would go green and thus speed through before the waiting pedestrians started moving forward on the same green light. All in all that day, remarked a reporter, the police had a busy time, "warning pedestrians that it was no longer proper to do broken-field running amid the automobiles."[10]

On May 20, all the 38 who received summonses the previous day appeared in court; most pled guilty. One was acquitted while the rest received suspended sentences. For example, real estate dealer Ivan Loren was fined $5, then had the sentence suspended when he appeared before Chief Magistrate William McAdoo and so passed into history as the city's first convicted jaywalker. Appearing for Loren was Charles Oberwager who argued the law was "trespassing" on the rights of individuals and was "violating the common law" privileges of pedestrians. McAdoo declared the city had the right to regulate pedestrians; "the common and statutory law from the beginning has recognized the rights of pedestrians for the use of the streets and highways, but it is not under certain conditions an unregulated right."[11]

Two weeks after that jaywalking ordinance went into effect in New York, and after all the publicity of the first day's activities, an editorial in the *New York Times* observed that, since then, "little or nothing has been done." Police Commissioner Mulroney, newly installed, had quietly rescinded ex–Commissioner Whalen's order to arrest jaywalkers on sight. Whether the ordinance was constitutionally legal or not was still to be determined by the courts, and in the meantime Mulroney thought it wiser to suspend "the hasty command" of his predecessor. To the ordinary observer, remarked the editor, the number of jaywalkers in New York City "has not been in the least diminished by Mr. Whalen's order, which was generally considered at the time it was issued to be ill-conceived and unenforceable." Concluded the editor, "By the time the legal question has been decided, the original order will have been forgotten, and no one will wish to have it revived. It is better so."[12]

In view of the publicity generated by the New York ordinance, journalist Myron Stearns commented on such laws nationwide. First, he noted that in 1929 there were 31,500 traffic fatalities and that motorized civilization faced a perplexing problem. On one side was a "tremendous" death toll from auto collisions with pedestrians, while on the other was "one of the irritating and often time-wasting remedies that is being applied on an enormous scale"—namely, the reliance on jaywalking laws to reduce the accident toll. San Francisco, Seattle, Los Angeles, practically all the cities on the Pacific coast, said Stearns, and a great many others throughout the rest of the country, particularly in the Midwest and the Southwest, were relying on such measures. Fort Worth, Texas, reportedly had been a strict no-jaywalking town for years. Other cities, such as Indianapolis, after a period of strict pedestrian regulation, had returned to a comparative disregard for rules about when or where to cross the street.[13]

Jaywalking laws, argued Stearns, were "directly at variance with one of the old rules of the road that gave a pedestrian just as much right to use the street as a motorist. The primary object of a street, according to the old English Common Law from which most of our own legal interpretations descend, is 'the free passage of the public.'" According to Stearns, such laws encompassed three points—speed, safety, and fair play. Motorists backed pedestrian laws because they thought auto speed was increased; pedestrians did not oppose the laws because they thought it improved their safety, but in forbidding walkers to cross a city street between intersections "such ordinances in effect give dangerous automobiles a right of way over harmless pedestrians, the third idea, of fair play, is usually quite forgotten." After looking at cities with and without jaywalking laws, Stearns declared, "If they prove anything at all, it is that pedestrian control has improved safety conditions little, if any." He concluded, "Clearly, most jaywalker laws for pedestrian control discriminate unfairly in favor of the motorist. Clearly, they waste far more time than they save. Theoretically, in the matter of safety, they do not really help."[14]

Another who had an eye on the New York City experience with the jaywalking ordinance was the editor of the *Saturday Evening Post*, who at first, and briefly, expressed some concern for pedestrians and no sympathy for careless and reckless drivers. But then he took another tack as he joined the antipedestrian legion by arguing there was another class of motorists who were entitled to much better treatment than they received from pedestrians or the law. It was a reference to the so-called careful and experienced drivers who, through no fault of their own, sometimes injured "foolhardy and reckless pedestrians who dash or move through vehicular traffic with no more care for their own safety than if they were crossing their own living rooms." Continuing his rant against walkers, the editor moaned, "No matter how careful and alert the motorist, if he hurts the most reckless of such pedestrians he will be arrested. He must get bail. He may face criminal charges, he may have to defend civil suits and, perhaps, pay heavy damages for an unavoidable and involuntary act. There is no justice in such a state of affairs, and no one pretends there is, but the condition is one that will prevail until widespread and concerted action finally does away with it."[15]

Arthur Blanchard, a Highway Traffic Control Consultant in Providence, Rhode Island, presented a paper on the rights of pedestrians, in 1932 at an annual meeting of the Institute of Traffic Engineers. He argued that since ancient times the law had been a haven of refuge for the pedestrian, recognizing in a tangible manner the rights of pedestrians; he regretted that most highway officials and traffic specialists had the idea "that it is only the welfare of the motorist which needs consideration." Also noted by Blanchard was that in the case of car and pedestrian collisions where contributory negligence was not proved, no recovery of damages was possible, and "There can be no recovery in the absence of negligence. Thus there is no liability for a pure accident," he declared. Agreeing traffic control signal practices had developed rapidly during the previous five years, he stated that "the pedestrian has been given scant consideration. He has been confronted, in many instances, with long intervals of waiting, right and left turns by motorists, and practically instantaneous changes from green to red with the waiting vehicular traffic starting immediately across his path."[16]

The UK's long campaign to get walkers to use the pedestrian crosswalks began in the early 1930s. During a 1934 debate on the subject, the Pedestrians' Association issued an official statement regarding the proposal to make the use of pedestrian crosswalks compulsory. The organization opposed the idea for various reasons: "It was an unreasonable invasion of the rights of the walking public"; roads were a communal possession and therefore all persons had a right to a reasonable use of them; and it would involve a very serious economic loss, far exceeding the economic loss resulting from any congestion of vehicular traffic. For example, such a rule would make it more difficult for pedestrians to visit businesses located across the road but not at the designated crossings.[17]

Over three years later, the Pedestrians' Association submitted a report it had produced to the UK Minister of Transport. It remained opposed to the idea of making it illegal to cross the road at other than pedestrian crossings. (The idea was still under consideration and still being debated.) In that report the group declared, "There is no doubt that it is the drivers of motor-vehicles who are mainly responsible for the installation of these crossings not having achieved the results which were looked for by their promoters."[18]

Due to the blackouts in the UK during World War II, the pedestrian crossings were rendered "useless" at night, with the result, said a 1947 news account, that there was a tendency for pedestrians and drivers to disregard them; a tendency that continued after the war and the blackout periods had both ended. As a result, local government authorities had begun asking the Ministry of Transport to support a new campaign to increase the use of pedestrian crossings and to get rid of an old practice that had returned — that of "dodging the traffic."[19]

Lloyd Rader was an American civil engineer, and in a 1934 issue of the trade journal *Civil Engineering* he observed that it was then the practice in some municipalities (such as New York) to grant vehicles the "privilege" of making right turns on red lights at intersections controlled by signals. While he agreed the practice expedited vehicular movements, he also believed those cars often blocked intersections and increased the danger to pedestrians, "thus one of the main objects of signal control at intersections — namely, the protection of pedestrians — is not attained." Rader was not alone, for the National Conference on Street and Highway Safety had formally placed itself on record as being opposed to the practice of permitting turns on red lights, except under special conditions where proper signs and signals were installed.[20]

Industry sometimes joined in the battle against jaywalking. A safety drive was started in November 1935 by the Westinghouse Lamp Company in Bloomfield, New Jersey, to remind its employees of the danger in jaywalking when leaving the factory at quitting time and at lunch periods. Although nearby street intersections were marked with crosswalks, the main entrance was right in the middle of the block. Several thousand employees swarmed onto the street from that main gate. Safety circulars were distributed to all employees using that entrance. On those circulars was a map of the streets around the main entrance with an indication where employees should not cross the street. All employees were encouraged to use the crosswalks. Large metal signs were erected by the police that told people not to cross in mid-block, but only at the crosswalks. From the plant employees, two monitors were selected to guide the crowd for a three-day period that inaugurated the safety plan.[21]

In an unnamed American city in 1935, an engineer methodically timed 60,000 men, women and children as they travelled a distance of 100 feet from one side of the street to the other. On the basis of speed they were sorted into three groups: the actives, the inactives, and the slows. Actives made up 84 percent of the sample and crossed the street in 20.5 seconds on average, or 4.8 feet per second. Inactives, 14 percent of the group, took 24 seconds, 4.4 feet per second, while the slows (two percent) took 31 seconds on average, 3.6 feet per second. Business reporter Gove Hambidge remarked that "any system of traffic control, to be effective, must give them every facility to move at their natural pace, exactly as in the case of other elements in traffic.... Too often the pedestrian gets scant attention." He thought a traffic signal length of 50 to 60 seconds (a full cycle from green to green) was about right for pedestrian needs and, as signal length increased, accident risk increased. With a 60-second interval, the accident risk was reportedly six times what it was when the interval was 20 seconds. "When the interval gets long enough, nearly everybody becomes a traffic dodger," he explained.[22]

Hambidge believed the movement to build pedestrian subways—tried in many places—failed because everywhere walkers simply refused to use them. Turns were another sore point for him, as he thought all turns to be especially bad in the sense of increasing risks for walkers (and he meant turns on both green and red lights). He even argued it might be necessary to curtail turns during the periods of heavy traffic. As another way to solve the problems of turns, he suggested a short period in the traffic signal cycle when all vehicle movement was stopped with pedestrians allowed to cross unimpeded. In Hambidge's opinion, the whole traffic problem was recent, with the first dedicated "traffic officer" in a police department only coming into existence in 1903 (in New York City). Electric traffic control signals had not even begun to develop until 25 years earlier, around 1910. Then, continued Hambidge, no great headway was made in that area until around 1924, with the first "progressive" traffic control system being tried out in 1926 in Chicago.[23]

In another of his 1936 automotive columns in the *New York Times*, James Spearing gave one or two lip-service lines to the idea that careless motorists existed before quickly moving to his real goal—to deliver an antipedestrian rant. "[I]n many instances of conflict between motorist and pedestrian it is the pedestrian and not the motorist who is the bully," he declared. They did so through their carelessness, deliberate or not, and therefore such persons should be protected from themselves by the regulation of pedestrian traffic. One who agreed was J. W. Frazer, vice president of Chrysler, who asserted, "Legislation has been aimed almost entirely at the motorist, and the pedestrian has been permitted to be as careless and unreasonable as he pleases." As far as Frazer was concerned, fining pedestrians for violating traffic regulations "is in no sense an infringement of personal liberty." He believed that when a pedestrian exposed himself to danger he was transgressing the rights of motorists. Frazer observed, "in some countries the pedestrian is considered in the wrong whenever he is struck" and, although he would not advocate anything as drastic as the assumption that the pedestrian is always wrong, "it is just as reasonable as the other assumption that the motorist is always wrong."[24]

New York Police Commissioner Lewis J. Valentine petitioned the city's Aldermanic Committee on Traffic in 1936 for the authority to arrest pedestrians who crossed streets in mid-block or who crossed against the light at intersections, the so-called reckless walker who had become a major factor in the traffic safety campaign. That request was but one step in a drive that year to control pedestrian traffic in New York City. A campaign of education and persuasion was planned for the thoughtless walkers. Violators would be arrested only if they failed to heed "persuasion." One impetus for the campaign came from the fact that in 1935 in New York City a total of 660 walkers died as a result of collisions with automobiles; that represented nearly 65 percent of the total of 1,032 people who were killed in traffic accidents.[25]

According to reporter E.L. Yordan, underlying the plans for pedestrian control was the new concept of the jaywalker as a menace not only to himself but to others. Police officials objected to the use of the word "jaywalker" at all, believing it had become a mild catchword suggesting a harmless, absent-minded, or hurried walker. Thus, they preferred to drop that word and replace it with the term "reckless walker" to designate all those who crossed streets in the middle of the block and/or ignored lights and/or the directions of a policeman at intersections. A police spokesman declared the reckless walker to be an "inconsiderate, stubborn fellow who creates a traffic snarl" and who "represents a serious menace and should be dealt with accordingly."[26]

Yordan explained there had been two large-scale attempts to regulate foot traffic in New York City—one during the time of Police Commissioner George V. McLaughlin, and the most vigorous one during the tenure of Police Commissioner Grover Whalen. Reportedly, that latter effort failed because the public had not been "educated." When Whalen initiated the citywide ban on jaywalking in May 1930, "the public at large resented the efforts at enforcement or jeered at them. The campaign finally was abandoned." Before a pedestrian-control law could be introduced, police believed, the public had to be made to accept it as a necessary measure, not as a move to give the motorist exclusive use of the streets. In compensation for his cooperation, continued the logic, the pedestrian had to receive assurance that he could cross with the lights without fear of being run down by a turning car. In that connection, said Yordan, "the ban on right turns on green, now in force at some intersections, is said to inspire confidence on the part of pedestrians and a willingness to wait for the green signal before crossing."[27]

Governor of New Jersey Harold Hoffman (having spent five years as Motor Vehicles Commissioner of New Jersey) wrote about pedestrian control in 1936 in the popular general publication *American Magazine*. He said the average American city was divided into two camps, "as much opposed in viewpoint as were the North and South in [the U.S. Civil War]. They are the drivers and the pedestrians." Hoffman pointed out those two groups were not the same as those who owned cars and those who did not but, rather, it meant those who were driving at the moment and those afoot at the moment. Some 67 percent of the 96,000 city traffic deaths in the U.S. in the previous three years were said to have resulted from automobile collisions with pedestrians. One reason for the division into camps, thought the Governor, was the "almost universal" confusion about the rights and obligations of the citizen afoot. What was needed, he argued, was the standardization of traffic laws governing vehicles and pedestrians throughout America. He recommended acceptance of the Model Code proposed by the National Conference on Street and Highway Safety. Prescribed under that code was that, at intersections with signals, walkers were subject to the same rules as vehicles; at intersections not controlled by lights, the pedestrian had the right-of-way. At all other points, such as in the middle of the block, the vehicle had the right-of-way. Note that crossing mid-block was not banned, though, under the Model Code. However, admitted Hoffman, "To be sure, it isn't possible for the walker to enforce his rights against a contrary-minded motorist. The motorist carries the heavy artillery."[28]

In 1935, remarked Hoffman, the city of Washington found that 75 percent of its traffic fatalities were pedestrians; then it did a study that purportedly showed that in 51 percent of the accidents the pedestrian was at fault. Surveys done in various American cities were said to have shown that, whereas five or six percent of the motorists would run a red light, from 55 percent to 75 percent of pedestrians would do the same thing.

According to Hoffman, five out of every eight pedestrians killed in traffic were guilty of one of three major blunders: crossing in the middle of the block; jaywalking diagonally across an intersection; or crossing against a red light. Los Angeles and Seattle were named by the Governor as being often cited as the nation's model cities in the enforcement of pedestrian regulations: "They first sold the idea to the citizenry. And they sold it so well that the visitor in either of those cities who attempts to jaywalk enjoys the novel sensation of having some citizen bawl him out before a policeman can begin!" Police in Detroit, Washington, D.C., Wichita, Kansas, and several other cities were said to have had much success with a program called "The Voice of Safety." Under this program, a police car with a voice amplifier and an officer was parked in the street. Officers in the cars watched for pedestrian jaywalkers and then spoke directly to the violator in a voice that could be heard several hundred feet away. An example of what was said was, "That woman in the plaid coat is taking a very foolish chance crossing against the light. You'd better go back to the curb and wait, madam. You'll live longer!" There were no tickets, no arrests, and no force involved in that program, "just shame."[29]

With respect to pedestrian regulation programs in general, Hoffman believed if a jurisdiction tried to impose such a program without first achieving public acceptance the program was almost certainly doomed to fail: "That's why I say that regulations must be psychological as well as physical. We need 'consumer acceptance' of pedestrian regulation — we've got to sell the idea to the community on the basis that everybody benefits by it." Yet Hoffman went on to note the pedestrians' chance of meeting death in traffic after dark was four times what it was in the daylight, when traffic was much heavier. In New Jersey, 85 percent of pedestrian fatalities on the open highway occurred after sunset. Admitting that side paths along highways for use by the walker were sorely needed, all the advice he could offer to those who did much walking after dark in the suburbs was "to arm yourselves with a hand flashlight, the purpose of which is to indicate your presence and position to the motorist."[30]

Discussing the jaywalker in general in 1936, journalist George Copeland declared, "For him no regimentation, no obedience to mechanical gadgets. If he can sneak across traffic when the officer is looking the other way, score one. The few seconds he saves in this manner may never amount to much, but he goes after them just the same." In Normandy, France, he reported, anyone walking along unlit highways at night was required by law to carry a lantern. Los Angeles was said to have discovered that its average pedestrian would wait 38 seconds for the light to change; after that interval, he moved. Minneapolis imposed a $5 fine on jaywalkers, while, when pedestrian control was first initiated in San Francisco in 1928, fines of $1 were imposed; 3,658 people paid a fine that year. According to Copeland, though, by 1936 there was "100% compliance" with the San Francisco anti-jaywalking law. Copeland commented that New York City had twice tried pedestrian control, once under Whalen and once under Deputy Police Commissioner Hoyt. In the latter instance, a red "stop" hand was illuminated on Fifth Avenue corners between 40th and 45th Streets and an amber light put up for pedestrian traffic. The trial lasted 60 days but was judged a failure because pedestrians paid no attention to the signals.[31]

New York Mayor Fiorello La Guardia signed the new traffic code late in 1936 that had just been adopted by the city's Board of Aldermen. Most of its provisions took effect 60 days later, in February 1937. La Guardia vetoed four of the sections dealing with control of pedestrian traffic on the ground that the public was not yet ready for a ban on jaywalking. One of the new provisions was that drivers in New York City would not be permitted any longer to make right turns on red lights, except on the direction of a police officer or by specific and dedicated directional signals. Declaring that the problem of pedestrian control might have been worked out in theory, the Mayor said it was "extremely difficult to enforce as a practical matter." The city's populace, he added, was not prepared for police regulations that carried the danger of imprisonment due to walking the city streets. In La Guardia's view drivers needed to undergo a period of training and subsequent elimination of bad habits before the city was in a position to impose the possibility of fine and imprisonment on those who walked the streets. Admitting the regulation of pedestrians had been successfully accomplished in many European cities, he argued that result was due to the power of government and the training and discipline of the people. "To try to goose-step or to drive into formation march the residents of New York City is a task far more difficult than it would seem in reading a regulation of this kind," he explained. "We are accustomed to move freely and naturally and would resent a police regulation which might catch the pedestrian unaware when he cannot realize the necessity of such interference." Concluded Mayor La Guardia, "I prefer the happiness of our unorganized imperfection to the gloom of organized perfection of other countries."[32]

It was revealed in 1938 that three times as many men as women crossed street intersections diagonally. That statistic came from A. R. Ellis, president of the Pittsburgh Testing Laboratory, in a survey of pedestrian and motorist behavior conducted as part of the Order of Elks' national safety campaign. Ellis also found that jaywalkers who crossed streets in mid-block were equally divided between men and women.[33]

Police and the Columbus Automobile Club set up informal voting booths in Columbus, Ohio, in May 1940, where motorists were invited to come and vote on various issues of concern to drivers. On one issue, about 3,000 motorists voted four to one in favor of arresting pedestrians who violated traffic laws.[34]

Again and again the problem of what to do about drunken pedestrians arose. Acting on a survey that showed 62.5 percent of all traffic deaths in 1942 were pedestrians, many of whom were said to be intoxicated, Los Angeles Deputy Chief of Police Bernard Caldwell, in charge of the traffic division, late in 1942, ordered motorcycle officers to take drunken pedestrians into custody. Motorcycle officers were to call patrol wagons to handle those inebriated walkers. During a special drive conducted from December 24 to December 27, Los Angeles police arrested 60 pedestrians for being drunk, 11 intoxicated passengers in cars, and 36 drunk drivers. During that period there were 11 pedestrian deaths. A second intensified drive, from December 31 through January 3, resulted in the arrests of 76 intoxicated pedestrians, 16 inebriated passengers in cars, and 34 drunk drivers. In that period there were only five pedestrian traffic deaths, and, on that evidence alone, Caldwell declared his experiment a success.[35]

One jaywalking incident turned ugly in Washington, D.C., in May 1944, when a police riot squad was called out to help four policemen facing a hostile crowd during an altercation with two Marines who had disregarded a police admonition against jaywalking. The Marines were charged with disorderly conduct and held for the Navy's Shore Patrol. According to bystanders, both Marines were beaten and kicked. However, the police said neither was hurt but three policemen were injured and taken to a hospital.[36]

Writing in the *New York Times Magazine* in 1947, Meyer Berger declared, "the pedestrian is a baited and harried creature, accorded certain piddling privileges under common law, but faced, at least in large cities, with new humiliations. The latest of these is pedestrian-traffic control." Such control, he lamented, had been in force for several years in cities such as Los Angeles, Washington, Denver, Buffalo, and Atlanta. In New York City, Police Commissioner Arthur Wallander was said to have served notice that he intended to try pedestrian traffic control there, "despite the fact that the New Yorkers have resisted such control for twenty-four years." According to him, Police Commissioner Richard Enright tried it in 1923, followed by Commissioner Whalen in 1930; both failed. As an example Berger gave of the difficulties involved in enforcing anti-jaywalking measures, he cited the five-block stretch between Times Square and Grand Central Terminal, which required about 22 minutes to traverse on foot. However, 12 minutes of that was accounted for in the six two-minute traffic lights encountered along the way. Another drawback to enforcement he mentioned was, "An astonishing number of city dwellers see the pedestrian-control plan as an invasion of Constitutional rights. They maintain it sets up class distinction between the motorist and the lowly plodder." It reminded Berger of an indignant letter to the editor back in 1924, which said, "Sir, must we countenance a return to the medieval status of the pedestrian, when any lord or noble had the royal right to run down any serf who came in the way of his mount?"[37]

Dr. John Thurrot, a psychoanalyst and psychiatrist who lived in New York City and had studied the pedestrian, had his own explanation of the pedestrian situation. He thought that basically all New York jaywalkers suffered from anxiety overdrive—"an inordinate mania for achievement, an overwhelming urge to steal from Time." Noting that New York City had a higher percentage of neurotics than other cities, along with the most ambitious people in the U.S., he added, "To these persons Time is an all-important factor. They must back Time to achieve their ambitious goals, and nothing—certainly not traffic lights—will stop them." At one time, related Berger, the New York State Legislature considered a bill that would have compelled foot travelers on public highways to wear lights from sundown to sunup. Four years earlier, in 1943, said Berger, Syracuse used "scorn" to promote pedestrian safety with the amplified-police officer program previously mentioned. Berger called it "The Voice of Doom" program and said that a typical called-out comment from the monitoring officer was, "There is an intelligent-looking citizen risking his life because he won't wait an extra second for the green light." Reportedly, that Syracuse experiment failed.[38]

Despite all its previous failures at implementing pedestrian control, New York City tried again, with an informal 1947 campaign. (No ordinance or law backed it up.) It was carried on at just three city intersections: Fifth Avenue at 42nd Street, Broadway at 34th Street, and Seventh Avenue at 34th Street. A police officer was stationed at every corner of those intersections—12 in total. When they stopped a jaywalker and got an argument, they handed him a leaflet announcing that in the first two months of 1947 27 people were killed and 532 injured while crossing New York streets against the light. One policeman stationed at the Broadway intersection complained, "When I ask people here to get back on the curb, they say, 'What ya goin' to do about it? Ya can't give me no summons.' And it's true—I can't." At Seventh Avenue, one cop commented, "In the first place, trying to stop jaywalking everywhere would be like trying to stop bookmaking—you'd have to put a cop on every guy in town." Those three intersections were chosen because they were major traffic bottlenecks. According to that officer stationed at Seventh Avenue, "Maybe things aren't any better for the guy on foot, except that he's alive, but things are certainly better for the guy on wheels."[39]

Washington, D.C., began emphasizing pedestrian control, wrote David Wittels in 1939, and was still doing so 10 years later. If a pedestrian started to cross against a light in central Washington, a cop waved or whistled him back. If the pedestrian persisted, the policeman took his name and address and gave him a traffic ticket. (Strangers to the city got off with a warning.) Over the first five months that method was used, pedestrian accidents in central Washington were said to have dropped nearly 17 percent; after the first full year of getting tough with pedestrians, Washington reportedly jumped into first place in the national safety ratings. South Bend, Indiana, started a pedestrian safety program in 1940, and in 1942 started arresting pedestrians who did not comply with warnings. By 1945 the pedestrian death toll was down one-third. As part of a coordinated safety drive in Wichita, Kansas, police photographers roamed the streets shooting pictures of jaywalkers. Then the violators were warned or arrested with the enlarged photos posted in the lobbies of downtown movie houses. After the first full year of that method Wichita's pedestrian traffic-death toll was said to have been cut by nearly 50 percent. Yet, the cause of pedestrian accidents often lay elsewhere, as Wittels pointed out. After noting that often millions of dollars were spent on traffic improvement with not a cent for pedestrian protection, he cited areas of danger such as trolley buses loading and unloading in the middle of streets with little protection for passengers, no sidewalks along many roads, cars blocking crosswalks, and right turns on red lights. Hartford, Connecticut, installed improved lighting on a number of its streets. During the year prior to the upgrade, 32 pedestrians were killed at night on those streets; in the year following the improvement, with the new lights on, there was just one pedestrian fatality at night on all those streets.[40]

The Broadway Association of New York City (comprised of business people, retailers and so on) recommended in 1950 a drastic curb on jaywalking, which it described as being a major factor in traffic congestion and as having widespread accident potential. It sent a letter to many other civic organizations in New York City urging them to join it in devising regulations against jaywalking. Signed by T. J. McInerney, managing director of the Broadway Association, the letter declared the group was "convinced" jaywalking was a contributing factor to the city's traffic problem and the group had adopted a recommendation that a local law be enacted as a means of curbing the practice. "It is apparent even to the most casual observer that the pedestrian who crosses an intersection against the traffic signal or who crosses a street between intersections invariably causes a slowing down of traffic and at the same time risks injury to himself and to motorists and other vehicle operators." McInerney noted that jaywalkers had "plagued" New York for several decades but asserted it was getting worse. A drastic regulation was an imperative, he argued, to protect "careless and impatient persons against the evil results of their ill-timed actions."

Despite his enthusiasm for yet another try at pedestrian control in New York, he did acknowledge that prior attempts had all failed, including the one in 1947 where leaflets were distributed at the three intersections. "Virtually no attention was paid to the warnings, and the leaflets only added to litter in the street," he explained. J.R. Crossley, vice president of the Automobile Club of New York, said the great increase in traffic volume during the previous few years necessitated the regulation of pedestrians. If that was done, he predicted, there should be a decrease in accidents and better traffic flow. "It is common knowledge that if people rush across the street when motorists have the right-of-way a chaotic condition is created. The driver has every right to expect a clear passage and often times runs into mishaps which are beyond his power to prevent."[41]

# 16

# Regulating Pedestrians, 1950–2005

> "Many traffic lights are rigged for the convenience of the motorist."
>
> Russell Davison, 1959.
>
> "There is no conclusive evidence to support the contention that pedestrian crosswalks and signals increase pedestrian safety."
>
> Louis Malenfant, 1985.
>
> "You know [New York City Mayor Rudy] Giuliani acts as if this is a city for cars and the people are getting in the way of cars."
>
> Fran Lebowitz, 1998.

As of 1951, it cost pedestrians in Los Angeles $5 if they were caught jaywalking, but in San Francisco, according to a news account, they had to pay with their dignity. That was a reference to the amplified-police officer program (mentioned in the previous chapter) that had been tried off and on in various cities, always apparently without success. When they least expected it, jaywalkers—"usually furtive female shoppers darting across the street from one store to another," according to this piece — were surprised by a voice that thundered something like this: "Lady! Yes, you in the brown hat! Nine people have been killed jaywalking this year. Don't let's you become a statistic." The voice belonged to traffic officer Charlie Bates, who each day parked his unmarked sedan outside San Francisco's big stores and lay in wait in the car for violators.[1]

Denver's busiest downtown intersection had a new traffic control system installed in 1951 that allowed pedestrians to cross the intersection in any direction, including diagonally. That dedicated pedestrian light lasted from 10 to 18 seconds, depending on the volume of pedestrian traffic. Advantages were said to be that, during the rest of the cycle, cars could turn right without being impeded by pedestrians crossing on green, and therefore not hold up any straight-through cars in line behind them. Reportedly, Denver officials planned to install the new signal system at most downtown intersections.[2]

Walter Gropius, in a 1952 speech at the National Planning Conference in Boston, said he hoped to see a revival of community participation of citizens, and "such a desirable trend could be best started by a campaign to recapture the right of way for the pedestrian ... while everything is being done for the car and its driver, the pedestrian has been pushed against the wall in the process of building up the great net of automotive traffic which has exploded our communities." Gropius argued that what was necessary were independent pedestrian traffic networks, "separate and protected from the automobile."[3]

In a 1954 editorial, *Life* magazine announced that, surprisingly, for the second year in a row the American Automobile Association gave New York City its award for the best pedestrian safety record of any U.S. city with more than one million in population. (This was in the face of most media reports that painted New York's pedestrian situation as one of anarchy on the part of walkers, and an ensuing poor safety record in comparison with other places.) In the editor's opinion, New York was one of the few American cities of any size in which the pedestrian was still free to walk "pretty much as he damn well pleases." In Washington — as in Chicago, Los Angeles, and Detroit, among others — if he walked against the red light a pedestrian might be arrested, and sometimes was, but "New York has no pedestrian laws." A seemingly amazed editor remarked that a New Yorker could cross a street in mid-block, or cross an intersection diagonally, or disregard a red light if he felt so inclined. Despite that lack of control the New York pedestrian had more chances of staying alive than walkers in most other cities.[4]

One of the earliest scientific studies of pedestrians and traffic took place in 1955 and examined the effect of high-status (clothing being used to define status) and low-status models on jaywalking behavior at a stoplight-controlled intersection in the central business district of Austin, Texas. During every 55-second signal cycle, the wait sign flashed for 40 seconds and the walk sign for 15 seconds. Subjects in the experiment were 2,103 pedestrians. In the control group, only one percent of the pedestrians jaywalked. When a low-status model set the example by crossing against the light, jaywalking behavior increased to four percent; when a high-status model led the way the jaywalking rate was 14 percent.[5]

Joseph Wepman, assistant professor of psychology at the University of Chicago, offered the following opinion: "Jaywalkers usually are people who haven't grown up. They still operate as if they were in the horse and buggy days. Man just changes more slowly in his own behaviour than his environment does." A psychologist (unnamed) at Northwestern University remarked, "I hate to say this, but most jaywalkers might be classified as personality deviates!" He went on to add, "Subconsciously they are seeking danger without knowing it, actually hoping to be injured."[6]

New York City opened yet another drive against jaywalkers in November 1957. That also was an informal and educational campaign with no ordinance or regulation behind it. Figures showed that in 1956, 441 pedestrians were killed in traffic accidents, accounting for 72 percent of all traffic deaths in New York; elsewhere in America that statistic was said to range from 26 percent to 30 percent in large urban centers.[7]

When New York City Mayor Wagner announced the new drive, he named Jack Straus, chairman of the board of R.H. Macy & Company, to head a 21-man Mayor's Committee for Pedestrian Safety. That drive was expected to continue through 1958, by which time, hoped Wagner, the public would be educated to practice traffic safety measures. No decision had been reached, added the Mayor, as to whether it might be necessary to strengthen the educational drive with an anti-jaywalking ordinance. However, Wagner hoped the city would not have to invoke such a procedure. According to Wagner this was the first time in New York City that civic, governmental and business communities had marshalled their combined forces to do something about the pedestrian problem. Police were instructed to call to the attention of walkers such facts as that they should cross streets only at intersections and only with the light, and so forth. Straus explained he had been sold on leading the drive by traffic commissioner T.T. Wiley, who convinced him that New Yorkers would cooperate in a "sensible anti-jaywalk program."[8]

Apparently that campaign failed, as had all the others before it, and in August 1958 New York City joined many other cities when it passed an ordinance making it illegal to jaywalk and banning the usual practices of mid-block street crossing and crossing intersections diagonally or against the light. On the first day the measure was in effect (August 8) police gave out 479 summonses for jaywalking, each carrying a $2 fine. New York police had, however, expected to give out many more.[9]

During the first week that particular New York City measure was in effect, an average of 241 pedestrians a day received summonses for jaywalking. Also, on average, 20 motorists a day got summonses for failure to give pedestrians the right-of-way. While the fines for the walkers were all for $2, motorists who interfered with pedestrians who were crossing with the light faced fines from $5 to $50. A spokesman for the Department of Traffic insisted "there has been a very high percentage of observance" of the new rules by both motorists and pedestrians. Traffic Commissioner Wiley, who had promulgated the rules, said that "engineering, education and enforcement in the proper sequence" had led to compliance by most New Yorkers.[10]

Russell Davison, writing in 1959 in a national magazine, voiced a common complaint heard from walkers since the arrival of traffic control that is still heard today. "Many traffic lights are rigged for the convenience of the motorist," he grumbled. "There are lights on busy boulevards where a pedestrian waits interminably for his chance to cross. When the light does change the time allotted him to make his crossing is infinitesimal."[11]

Around 1959, Winnipeg, Canada, installed the new Walk–Don't Walk traffic signals. Pedestrians discovered these new signals gave them only 10 seconds to get across the street; cars had the green light for 90 seconds. Thus there was a lot of non-compliance with the signals. People also wrote angry letters to the newspapers attacking the timing cycle of the new devices. After several months, city authorities gave in and extended the walk period, almost doubling it at the widest intersections. Following his report on the story, journalist Hal Tennant went on at length to explain why motorists had everything their way; for example, streets got widened and sidewalks narrowed, never the other way around. Motorists, he argued, always got priority in public spending while pedestrians never seemed to come first.[12]

Famed writer on American cities Jane Jacobs, in a 1961 book, argued against the attempt to separate pedestrian and vehicular traffic as being futile, and further said that any method devised to deal with the situation was doomed to failure unless there was a dramatic decline in the absolute number of cars using city streets. The real problem, she argued, was how to drastically cut down the number of such vehicles. Schemes that advocated removal of pedestrians vertically — down into tunnels or up onto overpasses — did not succeed because they provided very little extra space to vehicles. "The conflicts between pedestrians and vehicles on city streets arise mainly from overwhelming numbers of vehicles, to which all but the most minimum pedestrian needs are gradually and steadily sacrificed."[13]

Historian Lewis Mumford remarked in his 1961 book on cities that as long as the railroad stop and walking distances controlled suburban growth, the suburb had a form. But the motor car had removed the early limits and destroyed the pedestrian scale. It either doubled the number of cars needed per family or it turned the suburban housewife into a full time chauffeur. Mumford declared, "With the destruction of walking distances has gone the destruction of walking as a normal means of human circulation: the motor car has made it unsafe and the extension of the suburb has made it impossible."[14]

Nevertheless aerial walkways (skyways) did enjoy a certain popularity for a time in the 1960s and 1970s as a way of regulating pedestrians (and, more importantly, of course, to make things flow more smoothly for cars). As of 1970, they reportedly could be found in cities such as Cincinnati, Atlanta, Calgary, Winnipeg, and Minneapolis. One skyway advantage pitched was that they provided walkers with shelter from the summer heat and winter cold. Pedestrians in Minneapolis could then walk along seven downtown skyways linking 16 buildings. Four more were being installed to connect other buildings, and the city's ambitious plans called for 64 such bridges in 1985 that would tie together buildings in 54 blocks, while 13 blocks were to be joined by underground concourses. One of five pioneer architects to have worked on the Minneapolis system, Edward F. Baker, remarked, "With 514,000 people going in and out of downtown every day, it made sense to put people on second-floor enclosed walkways." City officials began studying a skyway system as early as 1958, recalled Lawrence Irvin, director of planning and development, but "people were so worried about what would happen to their first-floor businesses that we could not get off the ground." Eventually private developers built the Minneapolis skyways. As of 1970, 18,000 people a day used the Minneapolis skyway system, 7,000 a day in the summer.[15]

A study from the U.S. Department of Transportation in 1973 indicated that walking "could be a strongly negative experience and tended to be threatening to those who were most dependent upon it for mobility"— that is, threatened by vehicular traffic. In low-density suburbia, observed Robert Collier and Jonas Lehrman, sidewalks were often absent, and "In some cases, it has now become a status symbol to not have sidewalks or curbs."[16]

Around the same time, Arnold Reitze and Glenn Reitze argued that the lack of sidewalks in, for instance, wealthy suburban areas, "presupposes a dependence on mechanized transportation that may be foolishly specialized and unfit for the needs of a large portion of the population." Where there were sidewalks in America, they continued, they were generally considered to be unworthy of serious interest, and "We have all encountered the widening of streets, but who can remember having seen the widening of a sidewalk?" Additionally, the Reitzes argued the law of liability in regard to accidents was weighted in favor of the motorist at the expense of the pedestrian. Even if a pedestrian was the cause of an accident with a vehicle, it was the existence of the vehicle's force that caused most of the harm. Hence, it would be logical and fair to place the legal responsibility for accidents on the person who introduced the force into the situation, they reasoned. However, that was not so, as the driver was responsible only if his negligence could be shown. An injured pedestrian had to prove the negligence of the driver, and if he could not, he would not be recompensed. Prior to 1850 in the U.S., the general rule was that if someone unintentionally injured another, he had to pay, regardless of the reason. That tradition changed in 1850 in the landmark case *Brown v. Kendall*, in which Massachusetts Chief Justice Shaw declared it necessary for the injured party to prove that the person in charge of the offending instrument had committed negligence. The *Brown* decision quickly won near universal acceptance in America, to the delight of heavy industry and the railroads.[17]

In the mid 1970s, authors William Dean and Simon Breines argued that the time had come to end the auto's domination of city life and the unrestrained passage of cars in cities. Urging the adoption of measures such as street widening and the closure of some streets to cars, at least on a part-time basis, they declared, "Streets are too important to be left to the domination of the automobile. They comprise one-third of a city's ground area. At the present time most of our cities have little more than occasional pedestrian refuges scattered haphazardly."[18]

Researchers J. Curtis Russell, et al., conducted a 1976 study of the effects of modelling behavior on jaywalking activity. Russell first noted that a number of studies had shown that a model who jaywalked across a street could induce observers to do the same thing, but at a higher rate than for the no-model control group condition. This study tried to extend that research by manipulating the sex, race, and number of jaywalk models. All models used were classed as high-status (well-dressed in business attire); when two models were used, one crossed the street slightly in advance of the second model so it would not look like they were together. This study, conducted in Birmingham, Alabama, replicated earlier study findings, with its overall result being jaywalking by 48 percent of the observers for the modelled condition compared to 18 percent in the no-model control group. No differences were found for male versus female models or for white versus black models. A significant difference was found in the *number* of models, with 56 percent of observers jaywalking when two models were used versus 40 percent for the one-model condition. With respect to the observers who jaywalked, it was found the tendency to jaywalk was the same for male and female (48 percent, 48 percent) and for white and black (48 percent, 49 percent).[19]

Researchers Leonard Jason and Richard Liotta conducted a 1982 study that assessed jaywalking behaviors when the timing of pedestrian signals either facilitated or impeded compliance. As background, they noted that in 1975, 44,820 people were killed in traffic accidents in the U.S., of which 8,155 were pedestrians. Under facilitating conditions, the pedestrian walk signal was set up such that after pedestrians had crossed one street they only had to wait a few seconds before being allowed to cross the second street. Under non-facilitating conditions, each time one street was crossed, pedestrians had to wait about 30 seconds before being allowed to cross a second street. The site of the study was a busy intersection on the north side of Chicago. Across the 11 days of the study, an average of seven percent of pedestrians (92 of 1,347, daily range of four percent to 14 percent) jaywalked when they had to wait an average of 10 seconds (range of eight to 12) to traverse the second street. In contrast, 26 percent of pedestrians (338 of 1,305, daily range of 17 percent to 35 percent) jaywalked when they had to wait an average of 33 seconds (range of 31 to 34) to get the light for the second crossing.[20]

Starting in November 1984, and continuing for months, a series of a dozen or so two-foot by three-foot signs were erected throughout Calgary. Their purpose was to teach pedestrians how to cross the street. Under the legend "How to Cross Safely" were symbols depicting a standard three-signal traffic-light cycle. The words "Start Crossing" appeared beside a Walk signal symbol; "Complete Crossing or Do Not Start Crossing" beside a flashing Don't Walk signal; and "Do Not Cross" beside a solid Don't Walk signal. Calgary's traffic operations department began erecting the signs at selected downtown intersections when it became convinced city residents did not know how to cross the street. When traffic operations engineer David Griffiths was probed by a reporter, he admitted the whole thing seemed "elementary," but he explained there were scores of Calgarians who did not know what to do when confronted with pedestrian traffic signals. "It's an ongoing problem," said Griffiths. "Some weeks we get up to a dozen calls asking how to cross at traffic signals." Most confusion was said to arise when walkers were halfway across the street and the Don't Walk signal started to flash — turn back or complete the crossing? Fed up with explaining such intricacies to a baffled public, traffic operations manager Douglas Leibel suggested posting signs at selected intersections. Journalist Kerry Diotte reported that on-the-spot reaction from pedestrians was highly critical of the signs and "is almost always negative." Said pedestrian Myrna Johnson, "The city must think we're stupid or something," while John Howarth added, "I consider this a flagrant waste of taxpayers' hard-earned funds and an insult to our intelligence."[21]

Louis Malenfant and other researchers looked at motorist and pedestrian behavior at eight uncontrolled crosswalks on two streets in Moncton, New Brunswick, in 1985. The researchers noted that a frequent approach used to reduce pedestrian accidents at uncontrolled intersections had been to install marked crosswalks; however, "there is no conclusive evidence to support the contention that pedestrian crosswalks and signals increase pedestrian safety." And, they continued, it had been found "that special crosswalks tend to instil a false sense of security and that pedestrians will step off the curb and into traffic assuming that cars will yield to them." In this study, signs used to reinforce driver yielding were used and read, "Drivers yielding to pedestrians last week ____%. Record ____%." Signs for pedestrians gave instructions on proper crossing technique: "To Cross the Street —1. Extend Arm — 2. Place Foot on Street — 3. Wait Until Car Stops— 4. Thank Driver." Police were also on-site and gave out leaflets and warnings on the topic, but no tickets to drivers who failed to yield. During the baseline condition, the percentage of motorists yielding to pedestrians averaged 33 percent on one street and 60 percent on the other. Under the manipulated condition, yielding increased to 65 percent overall. During the baseline period, pedestrians rarely signalled their intention to cross the street on either thoroughfare. On one street, signalling behavior by walkers moved from five percent during the baseline to 47 percent under manipulation; on the other street, it moved from 0.4 percent to 5.0 percent.[22]

Brian Mullen and other researchers did a 1990 meta-analysis of studies (23,680 pedestrians were represented in the data) that all looked at the effects of modelled behavior on jaywalking, by observing pedestrians. According to their analysis, obedient models (ones who did not jaywalk) produced a small but significant decrease in the frequency of pedestrian jaywalking, while disobedient models (ones who did jaywalk) produced a small but significant increase in the frequency of pedestrian jaywalking. Disobedient models were found to exert a greater effect than obedient models. Crowded sidewalks exaggerated the tendency for a disobedient model to increase jaywalking and undermined the tendency for an obedient model to decrease jaywalking. Also, the status of the model influenced the effect of the model on jaywalking behavior. Specifically, an obedient model was significantly more likely to produce a decrease in jaywalking when the model was of high status [status being always defined by clothing]. However, a disobedient model was marginally less likely to produce an increase in jaywalking when the model was of high status. The influence of both disobedient and obedient models was found to be greater in cities of larger size. Under no-model control conditions, the average proportion of pedestrians jaywalking was 24.5 percent; that was decreased by an obedient model to 16.5 percent and was increased by a disobedient model to 44.1 percent. Nationwide, almost 20 percent of all traffic accident deaths involved a pedestrian; in the 1980s, that figure amounted to around 7,500 pedestrian traffic deaths per year. One study observed that approximately 78 percent of traffic accidents involving walkers occurred within 50 feet of the intersection; 40 percent happened within the crosswalk proper.[23]

Bradford Ketchum, editor of *The Walking Magazine*, said in 1990 that streets in many cities around the world might become less friendly to pedestrians in the future because of the dominance of the automobile and potentially harmful environmental conditions. He added that urban development in almost all cities around the world since World War II had emphasized the car — with items such as freeway systems, parking garages, and shopping malls catering to drivers and actually limiting access by pedestrians. As we moved into the 21st century, predicted Ketchum, pedestrians would find many urban areas to be "unfriendly," as highways would continue to separate destination from location, as car traffic patterns would continue to conflict with pedestrian movement, and as construction projects would block sidewalks. Pollution, such as increased ozone levels and higher concentrations of carbon monoxide, he added, would also make city walking "miserable."[24]

Mark Bricklin, in a 1991 editorial in *Prevention* magazine, pointed out the difficulties a pedestrian had in crossing city streets, as vehicles had all the power, all the speed, and all the lethality. As far as he was concerned, much of the major construction carried out over the previous 20 to 30 years had been designed "as if no one walks." As an example, he cited suburban subdivisions that were often surrounded by cornfields and major highways such that people could not walk anywhere. Bricklin told the reader that the federal government had just funded a project within the Federal Highway Administration called the National Bicycling and Walking study. Its director, John Fegan, explained the project's chief purpose was to tell Congress what needed to be done to encourage more people to use their feet or their bikes to get around. Bricklin urged his readers to let Fegan know their suggestions to make America more walkable.[25]

Some nine months later, Bricklin wrote a follow-up editorial on his earlier appeal to people to write to Fegan. He printed excerpts from the comments of a few people who did so; many complained about the lack of sidewalks—and safe sidewalks—in general. According to the piece, *Prevention* was then starting to put together a national coalition of community groups that would strive to encourage positive action for pedestrians at every level and urged such groups to write to him.[26]

Three months later, Bricklin returned with a third editorial, arguing for better and safer walkways for pedestrians. He said he had enlisted U.S. Congressman Don Ritter to help in *Prevention*'s new movement, which was called "Make America Walkable," and to call for a National Walking Week. Readers were urged to write to their U.S. Representative and urge him or her to support a National Walking Week.[27]

New York City Councilman Noach Dear said in 1996 that it was time to rein in jaywalking New Yorkers. To that end, he had introduced a get-tough bill despite a feeling among transportation experts that he was wasting his time. Vehicles hit 14,000 pedestrians in New York City in 1994, and killed 240 of them, which was well below the record pedestrian death toll of 374 recorded in 1989. Walkers accounted for half of all New York City traffic deaths.[28]

Next up in the never-ending New York battle was Mayor Rudy Giuliani. In 1998, after crackdowns on squeegee operators, litter droppers, and graffiti artists had made the place "the safest big city in the country," Giuliani turned his attention to jaywalkers. Barricades manned by police were placed on a few roads to force pedestrians to cross only at certain spots. After that, the Mayor took the campaign (but not the barricades) citywide. Leaflets urging "Pedestrians: share the road safely" were said to have only inflamed the atmosphere, as had Giuliani's labelling of protesters as "anti-car hysterics" and his rhetoric about cracking down on jaywalkers with large fines. While one of the mayor's goals was to reduce the number of pedestrian deaths in accidents, he also hoped it would lead to a faster traffic flow — average car speed in midtown had fallen to about six miles per hour — thereby boosting New York's economy. Transportation consultant Charles Komanoff commented that even if traffic moved 20 percent faster — as Giuliani predicted it would, thanks to his crackdown — the time the motorists saved as a result would be far less than the extra time pedestrians would need for their journeys. With many more pedestrians than vehicles crossing midtown, Komanoff speculated the time saved by motorists might be barely one-tenth of that lost by walkers.[29]

Commenting on Giuliani's campaign, author Fran Lebowitz remarked, "You know, Giuliani acts as if this is a city for cars and the people are getting in the way of cars.... The idea that gridlock is caused by pedestrians is a kind of Reagan idea, like that ketchup is a vegetable. Gridlock is caused by cars!" Appalled by his attempt to make "the pedestrian the villain," Lebowitz said, with regard to the Mayor, "I don't think he's nuts. I think he's evil."[30]

Well-known author and humorist Bill Bryson commented in 2001 that if you went to almost any suburb in America developed in the last 30 years, "you will not find a sidewalk anywhere. Often you won't find a single pedestrian-crossing." The fact is, he argued, "we not only don't walk anywhere anymore in this country, we *won't* walk anywhere, and woe to anyone who tries to make us, as the city of Laconia, N.H., discovered." In the early 1970s, Laconia spent millions of dollars on a comprehensive urban renewal project, which included building a downtown pedestrian mall to make shopping more pleasant. Esthetically, it was said to be a success, but it was also pronounced a commercial disaster. Forced to walk one whole block from a parking garage, shoppers abandoned downtown Laconia for suburban malls. In 1994, continued Bryson, Laconia demolished its pedestrian mall and brought back the cars. "Now people can park right in front of the stores again and downtown Laconia thrives anew," related Bryson, "and if that isn't sad, I don't know what is."[31]

Nicolas Gueguen and Nathalie Pichot conducted a 2001 study on the effect of modelling behavior on jaywalking activity in an unnamed city of over 300,000 people in France. Their results were similar to those obtained in America. In the control group (no-model) condition, 15.6 percent of the pedestrians crossed against the light. Under the condition of a high-status (clothing again the defining characteristic for status) model setting the example, 54.5 percent of the observers jaywalked; 17.9 percent jaywalked in the intermediate-status model condition. When a low-status model (unshaven; greasy hair; old sloppy clothing) was used, just 9.3 percent of the observers crossed against the light, an apparent inhibiting effect as the number was significantly less than found in the control group.[32]

New York City's Department of Transportation announced in 2002 that in the following months it hoped to challenge the attitude that jaywalking was part of New York City, with a public service campaign aimed at pedestrians. While the number of pedestrian deaths in traffic had remained stable since 1998 at about 200 a year, 11,000 walkers were still injured annually by cars. Transportation Commissioner Iris Weinshall believed the numbers would drop further if New Yorkers would stop jaywalking. To that end, she was working with city hall on a public service campaign that was to try and change the mentality of the New York pedestrian, described by reporter Katherine Marsh as "famously brazen." New York Mayor Bloomberg's campaign platform stated that walking should be made safer, easier, and faster. Commented Marsh, "But in a city in which pedestrians view jaywalking not only as a cultural prerogative, but also as their best weapon in a longstanding battle against motorists for control of the streets, the anti-jaywalking message is a hard sell."[33]

Marsh pointed out that in 1998, when Mayor Rudy Giuliani announced his crackdown and raised fines from $2 to $50, New Yorkers derided those efforts and kept crossing streets illegally. But this new campaign was to use persuasion. "If we can win the hearts and minds of people with advertising, that's what this country is based on," said James McShane, commander of the police department's traffic control division. One year earlier, the department of transportation asked Manhattan advertising agency Bozell to create awareness about the problem of jaywalking there. After interviewing walkers, Bozell senior partner Justin Harrington said, "There's city pride associated with jaywalking. We view people who don't do it as rubes." Not so in other cities, like Los Angeles and Milwaukee, declared Marsh, "where jaywalking laws are strictly enforced and pedestrians often wait to cross with the signal, even when there is no traffic." Charles Komanoff, founder of Right of Way, a pedestrian lobby group, thought the city had it backwards and that drivers, not pedestrians, were the culprits. In an analysis of police accident reports from 1997, Komanoff and his group determined that in 71 percent of the cases drivers were largely or partly to blame."[34]

Fred Kent, president of the Project for Public Spaces, a non-profit group that advised communities on public planning, saw the walking situation as part of a much larger problem, and said in 2002, "I think it is all part of this trend away from being comfortable as a pedestrian." He added, "American cities and American life in general is so focused on the car that we are becoming enormously obese, because we have few opportunities to walk and very few opportunities to exercise."[35]

A cluster of scientific studies published in August 2003 in the *American Journal of Health Promotion* showed life in the suburbs could kill you one way or another, according to journalist Tom Spears. It was dangerous to walk or cycle on North American streets, yet driving everywhere— thanks to the low-density urban sprawl city planners had created for so long, which precluded walking and cycling as options in many instances— left North Americans overweight and hypertensive. At fault, said Spears, was a tendency to base our society in sprawling areas where a car was considered a necessity to get around. One of the studies found residents of suburban areas with a lot of sprawl—big lots, wide streets, and a trip of several kilometers to the nearest store or school—weighed nearly 6.3 pounds (three kilograms) more than residents of more compact areas. Also, the sprawl-dwellers had higher blood pressure and spent an average of 79 minutes less each month walking. Poor accessibility was the common denominator of urban sprawl—nothing was in easy walking distance of anything else, according to the study of the U.S. National Center for Smart Growth. Rutgers University urban planner Reid Ewing rated the amount of sprawl in 448 counties that surrounded metropolitan areas, and then tracked data on the health of 200,000 area residents. All other factors being equal, each extra degree of sprawl meant extra weight, less walking, and a little more high blood pressure.[36]

In a parallel study, Wendy King of the University of Pittsburgh showed elderly Pittsburgh women (average age 74) clocked an average of 6,797 steps per day on a pedometer if they lived near biking or walking trails, but only 4,908 steps if they did not. Women who lived within walking distance of a department store or hardware store averaged 6,808 steps per day, compared to 5,015 steps for those not living near such a store. While more walking was regularly advocated, the catch was that North American cyclists and pedestrians were up to six times more likely to be killed in traffic than were their German or Dutch counterparts, said the scientists, because North American roads were designed mainly for vehicles. Per kilometer traveled, pedestrians were 23 times more likely to get killed in traffic than car occupants in 2001, while bicyclists were 12 times more likely to get killed than were car occupants, according to John Pucher of Rutgers University.[37]

# 17

# Conclusion

Through to approximately the 1700s, walking was something almost everyone did out of necessity. For much of the populace, birth, life, and death all took place within a very small area, the distance a person could comfortably walk in a day or so. Wealthier folks enjoyed a few more options, such as the horse and animal-drawn wheeled carts. As the transportation revolution spread throughout society in the late 1700s and into the 1800s, relatively cheap transportation became more readily available to people in the lower classes, which greatly enlarged the geographical scope of their lives. An offshoot from the transportation system changes was that walking became something that was done more and more out of choice, instead of necessity. Long walks, or excursive walking, became very popular in England and other parts of Europe in this same period, from the very late 1700s through much of the 1800s. Whereas books for travelers published prior to 1800 rarely mentioned walking, they regularly did so after that date. Giving the activity a higher profile and greater popularity was the fact that so many of the European excursive walkers were famous literary figures.

No such parallel development took place in America at that time. The United States was geographically too vast and too sparsely settled for walking to play much of a noticeable part in the nation's early history. But individuals often walked considerable distances in pursuit of solitary occupations such as fur trapper. After the Civil War, walking became a more visible and a more commented-on activity in America. Promenading became a popular activity in the larger cities and resort areas, especially among the bourgeois. While nothing in America paralleled the excursive walks of the European literary set — walks of a huge distance designed to induce contemplation in the stroller, and observation of nature, and intellectual creativity — a type of distance walking did emerge.

Its time was from the 1870s to around World War I. Filtered through the prism of American buccaneer capitalism, the leisurely, contemplative, observational European excursive walk became in the U.S. a series of races—competitions with prizes for the grim-faced walkers, who often went around and around on an indoor track, hour after hour, day after day, until, under a Darwinian ethos, they literally fell by the wayside. Such competitions often drew huge crowds of spectators, and walking heroes emerged to be adored by the public. The best-known walker was probably Edward Weston, who got a great deal of media attention. Besides the race participants there were various individuals who undertook huge walks alone (from New York to Chicago, from New York to San Francisco, and so forth), or in a competitive situation against one or more opponents. Finally, as lying and cheating became more and more a feature of American distance walking and as the sheer number of races weakened interest, the activity faded away. Over time, the fad of distance walking would strike America again, but only in a limited way and for a limited time. Most well known of those were the much publicized 50-mile hikes during the time of President John F. Kennedy's administration.

As early as 1900, observers were reporting an idea that would continue to be heard up to the current time — that nobody walked anymore. Walking in America still had a philosophical side, a contemplative side, at least in the first one-third or so of the 1900s. Debate took place in magazines over the merits of the country walk versus the city walk, over the virtue of an aimless walk versus a walk with a purpose, over the benefit of walking alone versus walking with companions. People who walked, it was said at that time, could be divided into two types: those who walked to be walking and those who walked to look at things.

During this early time and to at least around the mid–1950s, there were next to no articles about walking speeds, or about walking conferring health benefits on participants, or about walking being an exercise. Walking was viewed more as an activity that satisfied the participant's mind and soul more than it did his body. In addition, there were no articles that purported to teach people how to walk. That topic made about as much sense as articles that supposedly taught people how to breathe. Both were things that people just did — naturally.

All of that changed in the mid–1900s, slowly at first, but then rapidly from the end of the 1970s onward, as walking received a renewed burst of interest and media attention. Much of that happened as walking benefited from the exercise trend that swept the population beginning in the 1960s. For many who were bitten by the exercise bug but found the trendiest of the activities, such as running and tennis, to be too strenuous or inconvenient for them, walking was a logical choice. With the increase in attention to walking came a barrage of books and articles on topics such as how to walk — the assumption seeming to be that few people knew how to walk. It was part of a change in which walking became instrumental in nature and not an activity which itself could be enjoyed and savored.

Instructions were often so elementary as to advise women not to wear high heels when they went for a walk. There were instructions on how to swing the arms, how to hold the head, and so forth. Bizarrely, the warm-up period (with exercises) was added to the politically correct walk, and was soon joined by the cool-down period (with exercises). What had been the simple pleasure in the 1950s — or any time earlier — of opening the door and going outside for a 20-minute walk had been replaced by donning a walking outfit, lacing on a pair of specific "walking" shoes, doing 10 minutes of warm-up stretching exercises, then going outside with your heart rate target zone monitoring system and pedometer for a 20-minute walk, and then home for 10 minutes of cool-down stretching exercises. A pleasure was recast as a chore. Not mentioned as goals of walks were things such as observation, contemplation, or thinking. Rather, the opposite was the case. People were regularly advised to wear a Walkman or similar device, precisely so they would *not* have to observe or contemplate; people were advised to get friends to walk with them, precisely so they would *not* have to observe or contemplate. That is, an underlying assumption for all such advice seemed to be that walking was boring, that it had nothing to offer in its own right. The fad of indoor walking at malls had the effect, of course, of even removing nature from the experience of a walk.

As walking was rediscovered from the late 1970s onward, it was reinvented in many ways. Being treated instrumentally was one way. Another facet was a preoccupation with numbers, from the heart rate target zone figure to the calorie burn rate involved. In many cases, the mathematics presented in the popular media with respect to those concepts ranged from questionable to woeful. Over time, the standard of what it took to be defined as a regular walker was lowered to such an extent that, by the 1990s or so, a person was often defined as such if he walked just 60 minutes a week (at least three sessions of at least 20 minutes each). Such low standards would have shocked observers in the 1950s and any earlier times.

Perhaps, though, the lowered standard of who was a "walker," by enlarging the number of participants, made it easier for marketers to sell the walking paraphernalia — mostly shoes — produced in such profusion from the early 1980s onward. The sale of so many "walking" shoes when there had been no demand for them, and certainly no need, was testament to the likely influence of professional marketers in the walking fad.

Walkers became pedestrians whenever they interacted with vehicles, and when the 1900s began pedestrians had already been killed by cars.

More than any other single factor, the automobile was responsible for the decline of walking in America — as the population of cars increased and land use catered to the vehicle. Poor city planning, suburban sprawl, no sidewalks at all in many suburbs, and separation of living areas from shopping areas from employment areas by relatively large distances, all made cars a necessity and walking difficult or impossible. Every year, thousands of pedestrians were killed as a result of collisions with automobiles, yet rarely, if ever, were complaints made about the situation. Despite the fact that everything was structured in their favor, motorists tended to display various degrees of hostility toward pedestrians. While the cars contained all the force and all the lethality, it was usually the pedestrian that was blamed when the two met in an accident. Generally, police treated leniently motorists who knocked down pedestrians, even when the latter were killed. Pedestrians were regularly portrayed in the media as reckless and careless, authors of their own demise.

Because of the arrival of the automobile, official attempts were made to regulate and control pedestrians, starting early in the 1900s. A major effort, still ongoing, was to stop pedestrians from jaywalking. It was an effort that was presented as having as its goal the reduction of pedestrian deaths and injuries, despite the fact there was no evidence that traffic signal-controlled intersections or crosswalks reduced accidents. Rights of pedestrians to have access to the streets— once quite liberal — were eroded over time as more and more measures were enacted to make things go more smoothly and more quickly for vehicles.

Over the last century or so, the forces of American society have worked to limit walking by making it increasingly difficult. Those forces have succeeded all too well, as the more sedentary population, produced in part by less and less walking, became more obese and suffered more health problems. Yet anybody who fought that trend and continued to be a walker in the face of all obstacles had to contend with the fact that per kilometer traveled in 2001, pedestrians in America were 23 times more likely to get killed in traffic than were car occupants.

# Notes

## Chapter 1

1. Howard O'Hagan. "Why have we lost the joy of walking?" *Maclean's* 70 (May 11, 1957): 32.
2. "Greeks know value of the long walk." *Science News Letter* 70 (July 21, 1956): 37.
3. Simon Breines and William J. Dean. *The Pedestrian Revolution: Streets Without Cars.* New York: Vintage, 1974, pp. 12, 14.
4. Ibid., pp. 14-5.
5. Ibid., pp. 15-16, 23.
6. "Marching back to 1066." *Life* 40 (March 26, 1956): 161-163.
7. Lewis Mumford. *The City in History: Its Origins, Its Transformations, and Its Prospects.* New York: Harcourt, Brace & World, 1961, p. 370.
8. Bernard Rudofsky. *Streets for People: a Primer for Americans.* Garden City, New York: Doubleday, 1969, pp. 44-45.
9. Anne D. Wallace. *Walking, Literature, and English Culture.* Oxford: Clarendon Press, 1993, pp. 10, 20, 23.
10. Ibid., pp. 29-30.
11. Ibid., pp. 31, 33, 53-54, 65.
12. Ibid., pp. 166-167, 170-171.
13. Penelope J. Corfield. "Walking the city streets; the urban odyssey in eighteenth-century England." *Journal of Urban History* 16 (February, 1990): 133, 135.
14. Ibid., pp. 135-136, 150.
15. "The pedestrian's progress." *Times* (London), September 27, 1930, p. 11.
16. Howard O'Hagan, op. cit., p. 60.
17. David Scobey. "Anatomy of the promenade: the politics of bourgeois sociability in nineteenth-century New York." *Social History* 17 (May, 1992): 203-208.
18. Kerry Pechter. "The first walking boom." *Across the Board* 24 (July/August, 1987): 44.
19. "Go as you please." *Los Angeles Times*, December 25, 1888, p. 5.
20. "Cheap walking." *Los Angeles Times*, April 8, 1894, p. 2.
21. J. B. McCormick. "Old-time pedestrians." *Los Angeles Times*, February 10, 1896, p. 3.
22. "Graceful walking." *Los Angeles Times*, August 11, 1883, p. 3.
23. Millicent Arrowpoint. "A walking cure." *Los Angeles Times*, September 1, 1895, p. 26.
24. "Walking backwards for a headache." *Los Angeles Times*, September 23, 1985, p. 6.
25. "The decline of walking." *Los Angeles Times*, September 18, 1896, p. 10.

## Chapter 2

1. K. Schmidt. "Stroll for health, boogie for fitness." *Science News* 140 (December 21-28, 1991): 405; Gerald Donaldson. *The Walking Book.* New York: Holt, Rinehart and Winston, 1979, pp. 9, 25.
2. Gerald Donaldson, op. cit., pp. 140-144, 166; "Walk the walk." *Times* (London), July 19, 2002, p. 21.
3. Gerald Donaldson, op. cit., pp. 166, 168; "Shanks' mare." *New Yorker* 39 (March 2, 1963): 24; Murray T. Pringle. "Tried walking lately?" *American Mercury* 84 (May, 1957): 36.
4. Gerald Donaldson, op. cit., p. 163; Arnold Haultain. "Of walks and walking tours." *Atlantic Monthly* 92 (October, 1903): 491.
5. Charles B. Shaw. "Afoot in the thir-

ties." *South Atlantic Quarterly* 20 (April, 1921): 153–154.
6. Edward Sackville West. *Thomas De Quincey: His Life and Work*. New Haven: Yale University Press, 1936, pp. 68–69, 96–97, 107, 144.
7. Gerald Donaldson, op. cit., p. 162.
8. Carol Kyros Walker. *Walking North with Keats*. New Haven, Yale University Press, 1992, pp. 1, 5.
9. James Kerr. "Walking—and some of its famous votaries." *Cornhill Magazine* 154 (August, 1936): 241; Donald Culross Peattie. "The joy of walking." *New York Times Magazine*, April 5, 1942, p. 10.
10. "The walkers." *New York Times*, April 29, 1928, sec 3, p. 4; "Shanks' mare." *New Yorker* 39 (March 2, 1963): 23; Henry David Thoreau. "The joy of walking." *Saturday Evening Post* 273 (January/February, 2001): 66.
11. Hunter Davies. *William Wordsworth: A Biography*. New York: Atheneum, 1980, pp. 24, 114, 116, 289, 296.
12. Theodore Irwin. "Let's get our feet on the ground." *Today's Health*, October, 1961, p. 75; Gerald Donaldson, op. cit., pp. 140, 164.
13. Valerie Grosvenor Myer. *Obstinate Heart: Jane Austen, a Biography*. London: Michael O'Mara Books, 1997, pp. 104, 117, 168
14. Richard Holmes. *Coleridge, Early Visions*. London: Hodder & Stoughton, 1989, pp. 60–61.
15. Gerald Donaldson, op. cit., p. 171; Bernard Rudofsky. *Streets for People: A Primer for Americans*. Garden City, New York: Doubleday, 1969, p. 48.
16. Edgar Johnson. *Charles Dickens: His Tragedy and Triumph*. 2 vols. Boston: Little, Brown, 1952, pp. 209, 458, 466, 1056, 1058.
17. Hildegarde Hawthorne. "A passionate walker's pilgrimage." *Century* 112 (June, 1926): 119; Robert Esmonde Sencourt. *The Life of George Meredith*. New York: Charles Scribner's Sons, 1929, pp. 45–51.
18. Robert Esmonde Sencourt, op. cit., pp. 79–81, 89, 155, 218–220.
19. Gerald Donaldson, op. cit., p. 167; "The art of walking." *New York Times*, August 1, 1926, sec 2, p. 4.
20. Gerald Donaldson, op. cit., p. 163.
21. Peter Steinhart. "The joy of walking." *Audubon* 89 (September, 1987): 10; Charles B. Shaw "Afoot in the thirties." *South Atlantic Quarterly* 20 (April, 1921): 153, 159.

22. Joseph Wood Krutch. *Henry David Thoreau*. New York: William Sloan Associates, 1948, pp. 54–55, 138–140.
23. Henry David Thoreau. "The joy of walking." *Saturday Evening Post* 273 (January/February, 2001): 64.
24. Gerald Donaldson, op. cit., p. 148; "Footpath and highway." *Forum* 71 (May, 1924): 674.
25. Gerald Donaldson, op. cit., p. 118.
26. Ibid., p. 164.
27. Ibid., p. 166; Evan Thompson. "Walk the walk." *Canadian Banker* 101 (January/February, 1994): 10.
28. Lilly Dickson. "Walking, Canada's most popular exercise." *Foresight* 8 (May/June, 1989): 34; Elon Jessup. *A Manual of Walking*. New York: E. P. Dutton, 1936, p. 16.
29. "Bell beats Roosevelt." *New York Times*, February 6, 1908, p. 1.
30. William J. Gaynor. "The pleasures and profits of walking." *Independent* 70 (June 1, 1911): 1198, 1201.
31. J. Brooks Atkinson. "Sunday morning walks." *North American Review* 217 (February, 1923): 240, 245.
32. "Lord Grey advises British to keep their walking legs." *New York Times*, August 7, 1926, p. 1.
33. James H. Hocking. "Do you know how to walk." *Recreation* 36 (May, 1942): 114.
34. J. M. Flagler. "The walkers." *New Yorker* 34 (August 2, 1958): 37.
35. Elizabeth Nowell. *Thomas Wolfe: A Biography*. Garden City, New York,: Doubleday, 1960, pp. 199–200, 219.
36. Theodore Irwin. "Let's get our feet on the ground." *Today's Health*, October, 1961, p. 74; "JFK's pace corps." *Newsweek* 61 (February 25, 1963): 24.
37. Bill Gale. "Talking about walking." *50 Plus* 24 (October, 1984): 62.
38. David Groves. "Well-known walkers." *Good Housekeeping* 205 (October, 1987): 118.
39. "Walk the walk." *Times* (London), July 19, 2002, p. 21.

## Chapter 3

1. Joel Garreau. "Don't walk." *New Republic* 211 (September 19, 1994): 24.
2. William J. Gaynor. "The pleasures and profits of walking." *Independent* 70 (June 1, 1911): 1198.

3. "Walking as a lost art." *Saturday Night* 25 (June 22, 1912): 6.
4. "Footpath and highway." *Forum* 71 (May, 1924): 673.
5. Edmund Lester Pearson. "Walking." *Outlook* 140 (May 27, 1925): 148.
6. Hildegarde Hawthorne. "A passionate walker's pilgrimage." *Century* 112 (June, 1926): 118.
7. "The vanishing pedestrian." *New York Times*, January 1, 1928, sec 3, p. 4; "The vanishing pedestrian." *New York Times*, January 1, 1928, p. 21.
8. Mary Elizabeth Magennis. "A walker's manifesto." *Commonweal* 14 (July 8, 1931): 260–261.
9. "Topics of the Times." *New York Times*, July 25, 1942, p. 12.
10. Gladwin Hill. "Youths too soft, physicians told." *New York Times*, April 1, 1955, p. 29; "Young fella, walk — or wither." *America* 93 (April 16, 1955): 58.
11. "After hours." *Harper's Magazine* 214 (April, 1957): 84; Howard O'Hagan. "Why have we lost the joy of walking?" *Maclean's* 70 (May 11, 1957): 32.
12. Murray T. Pringle. "Tried walking lately." *American Mercury* 84 (May, 1957): 35–36.
13. J. M. Flagler. "The walkers." *New Yorker* 34 (August 2, 1958): 37.
14. "Shanks' pony." *Times* (London), April 16, 1958, p. 11.
15. Theodore Irwin. "Let's get our feet on the ground." *Today's Health*, October, 1961, p. 30.
16. Robert Thomas Allen. "Next ... automated people." *Science Digest* 53 (May, 1963): 40.
17. George O'Connell. "How to win in a walk." *New York Times*, February 3, 1980, sec 22, p. 16.
18. Jane E. Brody. "Personal health." *New York Times*, May 28, 1980, p. C10.
19. Susanna Levin. "Walking." *Health* 19 (April, 1987): 35.
20. Mark Bricklin. "Change your life with a walk." *Prevention* 47 (May, 1995): 15.
21. Bill Bryson. "Out of step." *Reader's Digest* 158 (February, 2001): 69.

## Chapter 4

1. "Long walk by Y.M.C.A. man." *New York Times*, August 10, 1908, p 3; "Reporter on a long walk." *New York Times*, May 23, 1909, sec 4, p. 1.
2. "Youth walks 475,000 miles." *New York Times*, May 8, 1911, p. 1.
3. William J. Cromie. "Walking for health." *Saturday Evening Post* 263 (March, 1991): 68, 71.
4. Edward Payson Weston. "Weston beats hoboes." *New York Times*, May 23, 1909, sec 4, p. 1.
5. "Weston and walking." *Nation* 89 (July 22, 1909): 71.
6. Edward Payson Weston. "Shanks his mare." *Saturday Evening Post* 119 (July 31, 1926): 23; "The art of walking." *New York Times*, August 1, 1926, sec 2, p. 4.
7. Edward Lamb. "Weston the walker made pedestrianism a way of life." *Smithsonian* 10 (July, 1979): 89–90.
8. Ibid., pp. 90, 92.
9. "Stop fake pedestrians." *Los Angeles Times*, February 1, 1914, p. ST4.
10. "Going for a walk." *New Statesman* 21 (April 28, 1923): 73–75.
11. "Telegrams in brief." *Times* (London), February 17, 1932, p. 11.
12. "Transition." *Newsweek* 1 (June 10, 1933): 17.
13. Meridel Le Sueur. "The sleepwalkers." *New Republic* 75 (August 2, 1933): 313–314.
14. "Walking dean." *Time* 29 (May 3, 1937): 47–48.
15. "City hikers." *American Magazine* 152 (November, 1951): 62.
16. J. M. Flagler. "The walkers." *New Yorker* 34 (August 2, 1958): 33–34+.
17. "Taking a long walk." *Newsweek* 55 (January 4, 1960): 24.
18. "Half entrants finish 5-mile walk." *Times* (London), September 25, 1961, p. 6.
19. "Pretty soon everyone was in the act." *Life* 54 (February 22, 1963): 72B–72C.
20. "Hit the road, Jack." *Time* 81 (February 22, 1963): 22–23.
21. "JFK's pace corps." *Newsweek* 61 (February 25, 1963): 23.
22. "Put your walkin' shoes on, Lucy." *Broadcasting* 64 (March 4, 1963): 74.
23. Philip Shabecoff. "Germans walk, and they like it." *New York Times*, August 15, 1965, p. 72.
24. "Tramp ends at palace." *Times* (London), March 31, 1970, p. 2.
25. "Coast walk by 25,000 for Shelter." *Times* (London), April 22, 1970, p. 4.
26. Alan Franks. "Oracle of the great out-

doors." *Times* (London), October 15, 1983, p. 8.
27. Lynn Langway. "America's foot fetish." *Newsweek* 99 (June 7, 1982): 79.
28. Nancy L. Croft. "Marketing." *Nation's Business* 73 (November, 1985): 33.
29. Kathryn Knight. "Cheat walks out of record books." *Times* (London), November 4, 1996, p. 3.

## Chapter 5

1. Arnold Haultain. "Of walks and walking tours." *Atlantic Monthly* 92 (October, 1903): 476, 481, 490.
2. "An object for a walk." *Spectator* 98 (February 2, 1907): 170–171.
3. "Walkers must be made." *New York Times*, November 16, 1909, p. 2.
4. "Weston and walking." *Nation* 89 (July 22, 1909): 71.
5. "Of walking." *Atlantic Monthly* 106 (December, 1910): 856–857.
6. "Walking as a lost art." *Saturday Night* 25 (June 22, 1912): 6.
7. Elizabeth Onativia. "Pedestrian's lot is not a happy one." *New York Times*, July 7, 1929, Sec 2, p. 11.
8. Madge MacBeth. "Women I have walked with." *Saturday Night* 27 (February 28, 1914): 25.
9. "The new walking." *Times* (London), April 1, 1938, p. 19.
10. H. F. Ellis. "Walk alone!" *Atlantic Monthly* 198 (August, 1956): 88–89.
11. Theodore Irwin. "Let's get our feet on the ground." *Today's Health*, October, 1961, p. 75.
12. John Kieran. "Out of the city, into the open." *New York Times Magazine*, December 6, 1931, pp. 12–13.
13. Ibid., pp. 13, 21.
14. Robert Sparks Walker. "Miles in the rain." *Commonweal* 20 (June 8, 1934): 152–153.
15. Mae Kelly. "Walking revelations." *Hygeia* 14 (July, 1936): 625.
16. H. L. Brock. "The gentle art of walking." *New York Times Magazine*, July 12, 1942, p. 14.
17. "Legs." *New Statesman and Nation* 13 (May 1, 1937): 709–710.
18. Hal Borland. "To own the streets and fields." *New York Times Magazine*, October 6, 1946, p. 24.
19. "Gentle walking." *Times* (London), March 24, 1962, p. 9.
20. Peter Steinhart. "The joy of walking." *Audubon* 89 (September, 1987): 8, 10.
21. Ibid., pp. 10–11.
22. Winifred Kirkland. "The wayfaring woman." *Atlantic Monthly* 109 (January, 1912): 132–133.
23. "Walking as a lost art." *Saturday Night* 25 (June 22, 1912): 6.
24. Madge MacBeth. "Women I have walked with." *Saturday Night* 27 (February 28, 1914): 25.
25. "How women walk." *Literary Digest* 99 (November 17, 1928): 25.
26. Mae Kelly. "Walking revelations." *Hygeia* 14 (July, 1936): 643.
27. "How to walk." *Good Housekeeping* 111 (July, 1940): 128–129.
28. Jeanne Lamb O'Neill. "Let's take an old-fashioned walk." *American Home* 65 (December, 1962): 14.
29. Rosemary Ellis. "Fitness." *Working Woman* 11 (July, 1986): 102.

## Chapter 6

1. M. B. Levick. "The confusion of our sidewalkers." *New York Times Magazine*, August 3, 1924, p. 6.
2. "Regulating pedestrians." *New York Times*, December 11, 1926, p. 16.
3. "Too many left-side walkers." *New York Times*, March 9, 1928, p. 24.
4. "Line sidewalks to effect pedestrian control." *Engineering News-Record* 102 (January 3, 1929): 21.
5. "Easing pedestrian traffic." *New York Times*, September 5, 1930, p. 22.
6. "Educating pedestrians." *New York Times*, February 14, 1933, p. 14.
7. Stewart Beach. "Pedestrian drift." *Atlantic Monthly* 211 (May, 1963): 114–116.
8. "Walk, don't run." *New York Times*, December 2, 1986, p. 34.
9. Marc Santora. "Etiquette by New York pedestrians is showing a strain." *New York Times*, July 16, 2002, p. B1.
10. "Keep to the left." *Times* (London), April 29, 1922, p. 21.
11. "Keep to the left." *Times* (London), June 7, 1922, p. 5.
12. "The rule of the footpath." *Times* (London), June 9, 1922, p. 15.
13. "Keep to the left." *Times* (London), June 13, 1922, p. 16.

14. "White lines for pavements." *Times* (London), July 3, 1928, p. 12.
15. Kristy Sexton. "The death of civility." *Sunday Mail* (Brisbane), February 16, 2003, p. 30.
16. John S. Watson. "Cross-national studies of walking in public places." *Journal of Social Psychology* 134 (February, 1994): 119–120.
17. William J. Cromie. "Walking for health." *Saturday Evening Post* 263 (March, 1991): 94.
18. Alan Devoe. "How to take a walk." *Reader's Digest* 34 (January, 1939): 74–75.
19. James H. Hocking. "Do you know how to walk?" *Recreation* 36 (May, 1942): 106.
20. Pete Martin. "How to walk your way to health and like it." *Saturday Evening Post* 214 (May 30, 1942): 19, 77–78.
21. "20,000 follow in his footsteps." *American Magazine* 135 (April, 1943): 127.
22. "How to walk." *Good Housekeeping* 122 (May, 1946): 156.
23. Murray T. Pringle. "Tried walking lately?" *American Mercury* 84 (May, 1957): 37–38.
24. Theodore Irwin. "Let's get our feet on the ground." *Today's Health*, October, 1961, p. 76.
25. "How to walk happy." *Better Homes and Gardens* 55 (September, 1977): 234.
26. Jack Galub. "Walking: the most obvious and natural sport." *Glamour* 76 (June, 1978): 124.
27. "Walk it off." *Mademoiselle* 85 (January, 1979): 58.
28. "Beauty & health report." *Glamour* 77 (April, 1979): 298.
29. "What your walk says about the way you think, work, love." *Mademoiselle* 85 (July, 1979): 142–143.
30. Abby Hoffman. "Walk your way to good health." *Chatelaine* 52 (August, 1979): 65–66, 68.
31. Gerald Donaldson. *The Walking Book*. New York: Holt, Rinehart and Winston, 1979, pp. 118, 146, 163.
32. Elon Jessup. *A Manual of Walking*. New York: E. P. Dutton & Co., 1936.
33. Laurie Johnston. "Walk, stroll, stride, amble, but do it softly and beware of tipping." *New York Times*, April 5, 1980, p. 21.
34. Jane E. Brody. "Personal health." *New York Times*, May 28, 1980, p. C10.
35. "3 months to walk your way." *Glamour* 78 (May, 1980): 102.

36. "Walking your way to fitness." *Current Health 2* 8 (October, 1981): 17.
37. "Walking: an exercise for all ages." *Consumers' Research Magazine* 65 (August, 1982): 29.
38. Joseph McLaughlin. "Walk your way to fitness!" *Mother Earth News* 77 (September/October, 1982): 79.
39. "Walk it off, run it off." *Mademoiselle* 88 (September, 1982): 232.
40. Mary Ellen Pinkham. "The best exercise of all." *Ms* 11 (May, 1983): 59, 61.
41. Bill Gale. "Talking about walking." *50 Plus* 24 (October, 1984): 62, 64.
42. Rosemary Ellis. "Fitness." *Working Woman* 11 (July, 1986): 101.
43. "How to walk off weight." *Mademoiselle* 92 (November, 1986): 220, 222–223.
44. Steven Jonas and Peter Radetsky. "Get in shape, go take a walk." *Redbook* 171 (June, 1988): 88.
45. Ibid., pp. 88–89.
46. "Walking into shape." *Forbes* 142 (July 25, 1988): 196.
47. Hal Higdon. "To your health." *Nation's Business* 76 (October, 1988): 81.
48. "Walking: the exercise of the '90s." *Ebony* 45 (July, 1990): 64.
49. Marian Sandmaier. "Hitting your stride at noon." *Working Woman* 16 (October, 1991): 104.
50. "Walk it!" *Good Housekeeping* 214 (May, 1992): 84.
51. "Take a walk! It's good for you." *IIR Focus* 70 (March, 1993): 1 sup InFocus.
52. "Walking: Rx for better health." *Ebony* 50 (July, 1995): 59–60.
53. Kevin T. Knight. "Walk your way to a better body." *Better Homes and Gardens* 74 (May, 1996): 98.
54. Tracy Early. "Test your walking I.Q." *Current Health 2* 24 (November, 1997): 20–21.
55. Carol Krucoff. "Can't get to the gym? Activate your life!" *Saturday Evening Post* 270 (January/February, 1998): 26.
56. Gary Legwold. "Take a walk." *Better Homes and Gardens* 77 (July, 1999): 119–120.
57. Deborah King. "Putting a swing in your step." *Times* (London), September 20, 1999, p. 55.
58. Christine Gorman. "Walk, don't run." *Time* 159 (January 21, 2002): 82+.

## Chapter 7

1. "Walking clubs are the rage." *Los Angeles Times*, February 5, 1908, p. 16.
2. "A league of walkers." *Playground* 19 (September, 1925): 315.
3. "Ramblers fight to keep paths open." *Times* (London), November 8, 1980, p. 3.
4. Carol Krucoff. "Can't get to the gym? Activate your life." *Saturday Evening Post* 270 (January/February, 1998): 28.
5. "A pedestrians' defence league." *Times* (London), June 20, 1925, p. 10; "A pedestrians' defence league." *Times* (London), June 23, 1925, p. 12.
6. "Motor cars and the speed limit." *Times* (London), October 24, 1929, p. 9.
7. "The Pedestrians' Association." *Times* (London), November 5, 1929, p. 9.
8. "Road-hog and jay-walker." *Times* (London), November 6, 1929, p. 15.
9. "How to cross a road." *Times* (London), December 13, 1938, p. 21.
10. "Closures irrelevant to railway crisis." *Times* (London), October 14, 1972, p. 5.
11. Nick Nuttall. "Minister backs protesters who bounce cars." *Times* (London), June 6, 1995, p. 6.
12. Ben Webster. "There's a new word on the street." *Times* (London), August 28, 2001, p. 5.
13. "Pedestrians' associations." *American City* 47 (July, 1932): 68.
14. "The right to walk." *New Yorker* 36 (August 27, 1960): 22–24.
15. "Pedestrian League." *New Yorker* 38 (April 7, 1962): 36–37.
16. "The pedestrian." *New Yorker* 39 (June 22, 1963): 20.
17. "Road signs talk in Paris." *Times* (London), April 2, 1963, p. 11.
18. "Citywide I.W.W. campaign." *New York Times*, December 6, 1916, p. 11.
19. "Walking to work commendable." *New York Times*, December 7, 1916, p. 12; "Walk to work week ends in 8-mile hike." *New York Times*, December 11, 1916, p. 6.
20. "Dr. Finley to begin drive for walking." *New York Times*, June 15, 1921, p. 4.
21. Vera Ayling. "Walking for pleasure and health." *Atlantic Advocate* 57 (August, 1967): 83.
22. "Walk Mile for Health day is saluted by the President." *New York Times*, July 1, 1973, p. 28.
23. "Arrested for walking." *Literary Digest* 45 (August 3, 1912): 198–199.
24. Seymour Deming. "Common footing." *Atlantic Monthly* 118 (July, 1916): 74.
25. "Gasless." *Saturday Night* 31 (September 28, 1918): 5.
26. "Shank's pony." *Times* (London), September 15, 1923, p. 9.
27. Edmund Lester Pearson. "Walking." *Outlook* 140 (May 27, 1925):148–149.
28. "Road-hog and jay-walker." *Times* (London), November 6, 1929, p. 15.
29. "Walking as a punishment." *Times* (London), May 12, 1933, p. 15.
30. "Walking as a punishment." *Times* (London), May 22, 1933, p. 10.
31. "Youth plods along on hiking sentence." *New York Times*, January 27, 1935, p. 27.
32. "Walking might help." *New York Times*, June 19, 1940, p. 22.
33. J. M. Flagler. "The walkers." *New Yorker* 34 (August 2, 1958): 38.
34. Peter Steinhart. "The joy of walking." *Audubon* 89 (September, 1987): 11.
35. Jeanne Lamb O'Neill. "Let's take an old-fashioned walk." *American Home* 65 (December, 1962): 14.
36. Robert Thomas Allen. "Next ... automated people." *Science Digest* 53 (May, 1963): 40.
37. Joseph Wood Krutch. "If you don't mind my saying so..." *American Scholar* 33 (Autumn, 1964): 496
38. Deidre Carmody. "More and more workers hit stride." *New York Times*, April 29, 1982, pp. B1, B9.
39. "Walking into shape." *Forbes* 142 (July 25, 1988): 196.
40. Taki Theodoracopulos. "Take a walk." *National Review* 45 (September 6, 1993): 71.
41. Jane Holtz Kay. "Without a car in the world." *Technology Review* 100 (July, 1997): 54–56.
42. Bill Bryson. "Out of step." *Reader's Digest* 158 (February, 2001): 70.

## Chapter 8

1. Arnold Haultain. "Of walks and walking tours." *Atlantic Monthly* 92 (October, 1903): 495.
2. Andrew Fenn. "The king of outdoor exercises." *American Magazine* 81 (June, 1916): 101; Seymour Deming. "Common footing." *Atlantic Monthly* 118 (July, 1916): 72, 74, 77.
3. James Kerr. "Walking—and some of

its famous votaries." *Cornhill Magazine* 154 (August, 1936): 242.
  4. Juliet B. Pickett. "The witchery of walking." *Recreation* 32 (April, 1938): 9–10.
  5. Donald Culross Peattie. "The joy of walking." *New York Times Magazine*, April 5, 1942, p. 10.
  6. "Scientist says long walk is best election antidote." *New York Times*, November 6, 1940, p. 14.
  7. "After supper." *Times* (London), September 26, 1955, p. 9.
  8. Carlos Greenleaf Fuller. "I walked a thousand miles." *American Mercury* 89 (September, 1959): 66.
  9. Jeanne Lamb O'Neill. "Let's take an old-fashioned walk." *American Home* 65 (December, 1962): 15.
  10. Robert Rodale. "Strolling down regeneration lane." *Prevention* 40 (January, 1988): 17.
  11. Joe Gibson. "On walking." *Harrowsmith* 16 (September/October, 1991): 14, 16–17.
  12. Stephen A. Kliment. "A view from the sidewalk." *Architectural Record* 180 (August, 1992): 9.
  13. Mark Bricklin. "Fix your head with walking." *Prevention* 48 (May, 1996): 25–26.
  14. Jay Walljasper. "Walk your talk." *Utne Reader*, November/December, 2003, pp. 6, 8.
  15. Roy Hill. "Walking the road to better teamwork." *International Management* 36 (January, 1981): 32.
  16. Sallie Stephenson. "Fitness walking for health." *Supervision* 50 (March, 1988): 10–11.
  17. John Lawless. "Country walks blow the cobwebs from managers' minds." *Sunday Times* (London), April 23, 1995, sec 2, p. 10.
  18. Dawn Gunsch. "For your information." *Personnel Journal* 71 (February, 1992): 16, 18.
  19. Rosemary Ellis. "Fitness." *Working Woman* 11 (July, 1986): 98.
  20. Tom Shealey. "Walk your way to superhealth and slimmer hips." *Prevention* 39 (April, 1987): 114.
  21. Patricia Edwards Bleyle. "Heavenly gait." *Ms* 17 (July, 1988): 24–25.
  22. Lilly Dickson. "Walking, Canada's most popular exercise." *Foresight* 8 (May/June, 1989): 35.
  23. John P. Wiley Jr. "Phenomena, comment and notes." *Smithsonian* 20 (July, 1989): 22, 24.
  24. "Walking: the exercise of the '90s." *Ebony* 45 (July, 1990): 62.
  25. Tracy Early. "Test your walking I.Q." *Current Health 2* 24 (November, 1997): 20–21.
  26. Gail Vines. "The feelgood factor." *New Scientist* 158 (May 9, 1998): 53.

## Chapter 9

  1. Bernard Rudofsky. *Streets for People: a Primer for Americans*. Garden City, New York: Doubleday, 1969, p. 105.
  2. "Do motor cars make us lazy?" *Literary Digest* 78 (August 11, 1923): 25.
  3. "Monaghan urges daily walk to keep well during Summer." *New York Times*, June 28, 1925, sec 2, p. 1.
  4. "Advises walking on tiptoe like gorillas to keep health." *New York Times*, August 4, 1925, p. 1.
  5. "Decides walking is no reducer." *New York Times*, January 5, 1935, p. 19.
  6. Paul Dudley White. "Walking and cycling..." *Hygeia* 15 (April, 1937): 321–322.
  7. "Walking is urged as aid to defense." *New York Times*, June 18, 1940, p. 14.
  8. George Weinstein. "Walking for health." *Hygeia* 22 (May, 1944): 344, 364.
  9. Howard O'Hagan. "Why have we lost the joy of walking?" *Maclean's* 70 (May 11, 1957): 62.
  10. Murray T. Pringle. "Tried walking lately?" *American Mercury* 84 (May, 1957): 36.
  11. "Walk, walk, walk." *Newsweek* 61 (February 4, 1963): 74.
  12. Alan Brien. "Afterthought." *Spectator* 212 (June 26, 1964): 866.
  13. William Fitzgibbon. "Striding, the most natural exercise of all." *Reader's Digest* 100 (January, 1972): 152–154.
  14. "Let's take (of all things!) a walk." *Changing Times*, 26 (September, 1972): 28.
  15. Jack Galub. "Walking: the most obvious and natural sport." *Glamour* 76 (June, 1978): 121.
  16. "Walking, a good exercise." *Changing Times* 34 (October, 1980): 50.
  17. Charles T. Kuntzleman. "Walk!—whenever ... wherever you can." *Vogue* 170 (November, 1980): 172, 176.
  18. Joan L. Lippert. "Walking." *Family Health* 13 (June, 1981): 20–21.
  19. Kristin Donnan. "Walk your way to fitness." *McCall's* 113 (June, 1986): 49.

20. Susan Zarrow. "Heal your heart with an easy walk." *Prevention* 40 (April, 1988): 22, 24.
21. Gale Maleskey. "Walk your way to good health." *Prevention* 38 (September, 1986): 38–40.
22. Ibid., pp. 44, 75.
23. Larry Tucker and Glenn M. Friedman. "Walking and serum cholesterol in adults." *American Journal of Public Health* 80 (September, 1990): 1111–1113.
24. R. B. Roth. "Walk to save your life." *Safety & Health* 143 (June, 1991): 87.
25. K. Schmidt. "Stroll for health, boogie for fashion." *Science News* 140 (December 21–28, 1991): 405.
26. Carol Krucoff. "Taking exercise in stride." *Saturday Evening Post* 264 (May/June, 1992): 14.
27. "Workplace walking benefits women." *USA Today* 121 (December, 1992): 7.
28. Evan Thompson. "Walk the walk." *Canadian Banker* 101 (January/February, 1994): 10.
29. Jennifer Chrebet. "More ways to keep bones strong." *American Health* 14 (June, 1995): 92.
30. "Study shows a stroll by elderly adds years." *New York Times*, January 8, 1998, p. A15.
31. "Brisk walking eases heart disease risk for most women." *New York Times*, August 26, 1999, p. A12.
32. D. Christensen. "Brisk step can reduce diabetes risk." *Science News* 156 (October 23, 1999): 260.
33. Julia Van Tine. "Go the extra mile for a big, healthy payoff." *Prevention* 51 (December, 1999): 48.
34. Christine Gorman. "Walk, don't run." *Time* 159 (January 21, 2002): 82+.

## Chapter 10

1. "Why walking does not reduce fatness." *Current Opinion* 73 (August, 1922): 234–235.
2. Gladwin Hill. "Youths too soft, physicians told." *New York Times*, April 1, 1955, p. 29.
3. Bernard Rudofsky. *Streets for People: a Primer for Americans.* Garden City, New York: Doubleday, 1969, pp. 106, 334.
4. Abby Hoffman. "Walk your way to good health." *Chatelaine* 52 (August, 1979): 22, 60.
5. Suzanne Murphy. "Walk your way to physical fitness." *House & Garden* 152 (August, 1981): 28.
6. Ibid.
7. "Walking your way to fitness." *Current Health 2* 8 (October, 1981): 15.
8. Charles T. Kuntzleman. "Perfect exercise: walking." *Vogue* 172 (April, 1982): 287, 382.
9. "Walk to work!" *Glamour* 80 (May, 1982): 100.
10. Lynn Langway. "America's foot fetish." *Newsweek* 99 (June 7, 1982): 79.
11. Jean Maguire. "Stroll into shape." *Redbook* 161 (July, 1983): 78–79.
12. Bill Gale. "Talking about walking." *50 Plus* 24 (October, 1984): 64.
13. Jan Sheehan. "Walking: a step in the right direction." *Saturday Evening Post* 257 (November, 1985): 39.
14. "Taking a walk." *Fortune* 114 (December 8, 1986): 10.
15. Srully Blotnick. "First you put your right foot..." *Forbes* 139 (April 6, 1987): 190.
16. Skye Wilson. "A new road to health: walk, don't run." *Business Week*, September 26, 1988, p.140.
17. Lilly Dickson. "Walking, Canada's most popular exercise." *Foresight* 8 (May/June, 1989): 34–35.
18. "These shoes are made for walking." *Consumer Reports* 55 (February, 1990): 88.
19. "Walk it." *Good Housekeeping* 214 (May, 1992): 79+.
20. "Walking shoes." *Consumer Reports* 58 (July, 1993): 420–422.
21. Mark Bricklin. "Change your life with a walk." *Prevention* 47 (May, 1995): 15–16, 132.
22. Kevin T. Knight. "Walk your way to a better body." *Better Homes and Gardens* 70 (May, 1996): 92, 96.
23. Gerald Donaldson. *The Walking Book.* New York: Holt, Rinehart and Winston, 1979, p. 45.
24. "Beauty & health report." *Glamour* 77 (April, 1979): 298.
25. Abby Hoffman. "Walk your way to good health." *Chatelaine* 52 (August, 1979): 69.
26. Jane Brody. "Personal health." *New York Times*, May 28, 1980, p. C10.
27. "Walking your way to fitness." *Current Health 2* 8 (October, 1981): 16.
28. Carol Krucoff. "Taking exercise in stride." *Saturday Evening Post* 264 (May/June, 1992): 14; "Take a walk! It's good for

you." *HR Focus* 70 (March, 1993): 1 sup In-Focus.
29. "Walking shoes." *Consumer Reports* 58 (July, 1993): 424; Daryn Eller. "The world's easiest workout." *McCall's* 122 (March, 1995): 60; Kevin T. Knight. "Walk your way to a better body." *Better Homes and Gardens* 74 (May, 1996): 92.
30. Mary Ellen Pinkham. "The best exercise of all." *Ms* 11 (May, 1983): 61.
31. Anastasia Toufexis. "Make way for the mall walkers." *Time* 127 (May 26, 1986): 65.
32. Lewis A. Spalding. "Take a fast walk!" *Stores* 68 (July, 1986): 29.
33. Robert Reinhold. "Making healthful strides at area shopping malls." *New York Times*, August 13, 1986, pp. C1, C8.
34. William Stockton. "Circling the malls to get in shape." *New York Times*, February 8, 1988, p. C11.
35. Joseph Pereira. "Love blooms in the aisles." *Saturday Evening Post* 261 (September, 1989): 54–55.
36. "Where will we walk in the future?" *Futurist* 24 (November/December, 1990): 42.

## Chapter 11

1. Mary Ellen Pinkham. "The best exercise of all." *Ms* 11 (May, 1983): 144.
2. "And now ... the walking craze." *Marketing & Media Decisions* 21 (March, 1986): 10.
3. Judann Dagnoli. "Walking shoes may open gait to big profits." *Advertising Age* 57 (July 7, 1986): 12.
4. Ibid., pp. 12, 57.
5. Lewis A. Spalding. "Take a fast walk." *Stores* 68 (July, 1986): 25.
6. Ibid., pp. 26–27, 29.
7. "Taking a walk." *Fortune* 114 (December 8, 1986): 10.
8. Carol Hall. "Stalking walking." *Marketing & Media Decisions* 21 (November, 1986): 74–75.
9. Ibid., p. 75.
10. Ibid., p. 78.
11. Ibid., pp. 78, 80.
12. William E. Geist. "A new approach to fitness chic: learning to walk." *New York Times*, February 25, 1987, p. B1.
13. Ibid.
14. Susanna Levin. "Walking." *Health* 19 (April, 1987): 30.

15. Glenn Collins. "In fitness stakes, walking forges ahead." *New York Times*, May 25, 1987, p. 14.
16. Kerry Pechter. "These shoes are made for walking." *Across The Board* 24 (July/August, 1987): 38, 40.
17. Ibid., p. 40.
18. Ibid., pp. 40–41.
19. Ibid., pp. 41–42.
20. Ibid., p. 42.
21. Ibid.
22. Ibid., pp. 42–43.
23. Ibid., pp. 43, 45.
24. Ibid., p. 45
25. Ibid., p. 46.
26. Ibid.
27. Tim Megyesy. "Reaching the fitness-walking buff through lifestyle marketing plan." *Marketing* 22 (February 15, 1988): 12.
28. Ibid.
29. "Gizmos and gadgets for walkers." *Prevention* 44 (June, 1992): 97–98+.
30. Ian Austen. "Tracking your fitness, every step of the way." *New York Times*, September 20, 2001, p. C1.
31. Adam Nathan. "These shoes were made for talking." *Sunday Times* (London), January 9, 2000, sec 1, p. 5.

## Chapter 12

1. "Walking and character." *Los Angeles Times*, March 21, 1915, sec 5, p. 13.
2. "The telltale walk." *Human Behavior* 7 (May, 1978): 41.
3. "What your walk says about the way you think, work, love." *Mademoiselle* 85 (July, 1979): 141+.
4. Christopher T. Cory. "Daydreams in Manhattan." *Psychology Today* 15 (August, 1981): 16.
5. Deborah E. Perlmutter and James H. Perryman. "How to turn your plain old ordinary walk into something sexy, assertive or athletic." *Glamour* 79 (August, 1981): 102.
6. Sarah Vandershaf. "A happy pace." *Psychology Today* 21 (January, 1987): 68.
7. Holly Hall. "Tired? Take a walk." *Psychology Today* 21 (May, 1987): 18.
8. Joann M. Montepare, Sabra B. Goldstein, and Annmarie Clausen. "The identification of emotions from gait information." *Journal of Nonverbal Behavior* 11 (Spring, 1987): 33–35.
9. Robert E. Thayer. "Energy walks." *Psychology Today* 22 (October, 1988): 12–13.

10. D. Jim Walmsley and Gareth J. Lewis. "The pace of pedestrian flow in cities." *Environment and Behavior* 21 (March, 1989): 123, 131.
11. Helen Fisher. "The way you walk that walk..." *Health* (New York, N.Y.) 21 (September, 1989): 53–54.
12. Ibid., p. 55.
13. Ibid., p. 54.
14. "How, when and why you walk." *Glamour* 90 (August, 1992): 234.
15. Nancy Stedman. "Learning to put the best shoe forward." *New York Times*, October 27, 1998, p. F8.
16. Duncan Graham-Rowe. "Tripped up." *New Scientist* 164 (December 4, 1999): 18.
17. Hope Cristol. "Walking: a new step for security." *Futurist* 37 (January/February, 2003): 6.
18. Rebecca E. Lee. "A prospective analysis of the relationship between walking and mood in sedentary ethnic minority women." *Women & Health* 32 (no. 4, 2001): 1–6.

## Chapter 13

1. C. N. Holmes. "What walking comes to." *Scientific American* 121 (October 4, 1919): 335.
2. "Our eight-mile daily hike." *Literary Digest* 94 (August 27, 1927): 24.
3. "Housewives walk 3,000 miles a year in own homes, survey finds." *New York Times*, September 8, 1936, p. 29.
4. "Some startling figures." *New York Times*, September 9, 1936, p. 26.
5. "Shopper's walk put at 8½ miles a day." *New York Times*, October 27, 1954, p. 32.
6. Robert Lindsey. "Once upon a time, everybody walked to work; many still do." *New York Times*, November 13, 1972, p. 39.
7. Ibid.
8. Carter B. Horsley. "Ways of city walker detailed in study." *New York Times*, January 11, 1975, sec 8, p. 5.
9. Boyce Rensberger. "Pace of city life found 2.8 feet per second faster." *New York Times*, February 29, 1976, p. 46.
10. Deidre Carmody. "More and more workers hit stride." *New York Times*, April 29, 1982, pp. B1, B9.
11. "Walking: an exercise for all ages." *Consumers' Research Magazine* 65 (August, 1982): 28.
12. "Walking: the exercise of the '90s." *Ebony* 45 (July, 1990): 60.
13. Paul Z. Siegal, Robert M. Brackbill and Gregory W. Heath. "The epidemiology of walking for exercise: implications for promoting activity among sedentary groups." *American Journal of Public Health* 85 (May, 1995): 706.
14. Ibid., pp. 707–708.
15. "Hoofing it in America." *American Demographics* 18 (September, 1996): 31.
16. Jack L. Nasar and Kym M. Jones. "Landscapes of fear and stress." *Environment and Behavior* 29 (May, 1997): 291.
17. John O'Neill. "Some streets are made for walking." *New York Times*, July 23, 2002, p. F5.
18. Samantha Grice. "The pedometer test." *National Post*, December 11, 2002, pp. B1–B2.

## Chapter 14

1. "Walking is a dangerous occupation." *Los Angeles Times*, December 16, 1923, sec 4, p. 12.
2. William J. Dean and Simon Breines. "Footpower in the cities." *Nation* 221 (September 27, 1975): 271.
3. "A new-made class distinction." *New York Times*, July 11, 1925, p. 10.
4. "Fining the victims." *New York Times*, September 5, 1929, p. 28.
5. "Bayonets for pedestrians." *New Statesman* 36 (January 17, 1931): 432–433.
6. R. E. Simpson. "Pedestrian accidents." *Safety Engineering* 64 (December, 1932): 260.
7. Arthur H. Blanchard. "Have pedestrians legal rights?" *Civil Engineering* 3 (May, 1933): 269–271.
8. "Poorly planned highways." *Saturday Evening Post* 206 (March 3, 1934): 22.
9. "Stepping into the beyond." *Chatelaine* 10 (February, 1937): 51.
10. James O. Spearing. "At the wheel." *New York Times*, May 24, 1936, sec 10, p. 6.
11. "Now a clinic to teach pedestrians how to live." *Science News Letter* 34 (August 27, 1938): 141-2.
12. "Our point of view." *Scientific American* 160 (March, 1939): 132.
13. David G. Wittels. "They ask to be killed." *Saturday Evening Post* 221 (January 1, 1949): 11–12.
14. Ibid., p. 12.

15. "After hours." *Harper's Magazine* 214 (April, 1957): 84–85.
16. Lois Balcom. "The best hope for our big cities." *Reporter* 17 (October 3, 1957): 19–23.
17. "No place for children." *Economist* 244 (August 26, 1972): 22.
18. Susan P. Baker. "The man in the street: a tale of two cities." *American Journal of Public Health* 65 (May, 1975): 524.
19. Ibid., pp. 524–525.
20. Ibid., p. 525.
21. "Pedestrians, our self-endangered species." *Changing Times* 33 (March, 1979): 18–19.
22. "Heroes." *New Yorker* 58 (October 25, 1982): 40–41.
23. William Holly White. "The gifted pedestrian." *Ekistics* 51 (May/June, 1984): 224–225.
24. Daniel Charles Ross. "Doin' the pedestrian two-step." *Motor Trend* 39 (September, 1987): 116.
25. Eric P. Nash. "Don't walk." *New York Times Magazine*, August 29, 1993, p. 66.
26. Gabriel Shapiro. "Watch out for drunk pedestrians." *Safety & Health* 148 (December, 1993): 100–103.
27. Jay Walljasper. "Mean streets." *Utne Reader*, January/February, 1994, pp. 36, 38.
28. Ibid.
29. Robert C. Yeager. "Walk at your own risk." *Reader's Digest* 148 (March, 1996): 188.
30. Ibid., pp. 188, 191–192.
31. "Report reveals worst American cities for pedestrian safety." *Jet* 91 (April 28, 1997): 24–25.
32. Alan Thein Durning. "Pedestrian paradise." *Sierra* 82 (May/June, 1997): 38–39.
33. "Watch your step!" *Economist* 348 (August 15, 1998): 22–23.
34. Jess Minerd. "Protecting pedestrians." *Futurist* 33 (August/September, 1999): 13.
35. Gregg Easterbrook. "Street sign." *New Republic* 224 (March 26, 2001): 42.
36. Zosia Kmietowicz. "UK government urged to establish a national walking strategy." *British Medical Journal* 323 (July 7, 2001): 7.
37. "War on the roads." *British Medical Journal* 324 (May 11, 2002): 1107.

## Chapter 15

1. "Futile jaywalking." *Engineering News-Record* 97 (October 21, 1926): 649.
2. "Walkers are human beings." *New York Times*, December 13, 1926, p. 20.
3. "Oakland protects the pedestrian in its new traffic control." *Electrical West* 58 (May, 1927): 271.
4. E. B. Lefferts. "Effective regulation of pedestrians." *American City* 37 (October, 1927): 434, 436.
5. "Pedestrian traffic — regulation and enforcement." *American City* 36 (June, 1927): 789–799.
6. J. Haslett Bell. "The pedestrian and the city plan." *Annals of the American Academy of Political and Social Science* 133 (September, 192): 208–210.
7. Foster Ware. "'What good are rights?' cries the pedestrian." *New York Times Magazine*, March 18, 1928, p. 2.
8. Lewis Nichols. "The light for pedestrians." *New York Times Magazine*, April 13, 1930, p. 16.
9. "Jaywalking ban in effect at 8 a.m. today." *New York Times*, May 19, 1930, p. 1.
10. "16 jaywalkers get tickets in first day." *New York Times*, May 20, 1930, pp. 1, 12.
11. "Jaywalker guilty." *New York Times*, May 21, 1930, p. 29.
12. "A respite for jaywalkers." *New York Times*, June 2, 1930, p. 20.
13. Myron M. Stearns. "Your right to cross the street." *Outlook and Independent* 155 (May 14, 1930): 50.
14. Ibid., pp. 52–53, 80.
15. "The jaywalker menace." *Saturday Evening Post* 202 (June 28, 1930): 28.
16. Arthur B. Blanchard. "The rights of pedestrians." *American City* 47 (November, 1932): 85.
17. "Pedestrians and compulsion." *Times* (London), October 2, 1934, p. 11.
18. "Safety on the roads." *Times* (London), January 22, 1938, p. 7.
19. "Crossings for pedestrians." *Times* (London), December 10, 1947, p. 2.
20. Lloyd F. Rader. "The law of the road — traffic rights of way." *Civil Engineering* 4 (October, 1934): 517.
21. "Employees warned against jay-walking." *Safety Engineering* 70 (December, 1935): 232.
22. Gove Hambidge. "Pity the poor pedestrian." *Transit Journal* 79 (June, 1935): 173.
23. Ibid., pp. 174–175.
24. James O. Spearing. "At the wheel." *New York Times*, January 5, 1936, sec 10, p. 6.
25. E. L. Yordan. "For pedestrian control." *New York Times*, July 12, 1936, sec 10, p. 11.

26. Ibid.
27. Ibid.
28. Harold Hoffman. "Trouble afoot." *America Magazine* 121 (February, 1936): 40–41.
29. Ibid., pp. 41, 157.
30. Ibid., pp. 157–158.
31. George H. Copeland. "A curb for the jaywalker." *New York Times*, November 22, 1936, sec 8, pp. 12, 17.
32. "Mayor signs new traffic code, but rejects ban on jaywalking." *New York Times*, December 23, 1936, pp. 1–2.
33. "Men jay-walkers thrice as numerous as women." *Science News Letter* 33 (April 16, 1938): 252.
34. "Favor arrest of jay-walkers." *New York Times*, May 25, 1940, p. 18.
35. "Drive started on pedestrians." *Los Angeles Times*, January 5, 1943, p. 2.
36. "2 Marines, police clash." *New York Times*, May 7, 1944, p. 7.
37. Meyer Berger. "Footnotes on the pedestrians." *New York Times Magazine*, January 26, 1947, p. 18.
38. Ibid., p. 48.
39. "The talk of the town." *New Yorker* 23 (May 31, 1947): 17–18.
40. David G. Wittels. "They ask to be killed." *Saturday Evening Post* 221 (January 1, 1949): 65–66.
41. Bert Pierce. "Fining or jailing of jaywalkers urged by Broadway Association." *New York Times*, May 17, 1950, pp. 29, 50.

## Chapter 16

1. "Speaking of pictures." *Life* 31 (October 29, 1951): 16–17.
2. "Pedestrians get right of every which way." *Business Week*, January 5, 1952, p. 20.
3. "To recapture the right-of-way for pedestrians." *American City* 68 (January, 1953): 127.
4. "Through traffic." *Life* 37 (November 1, 1954): 30.
5. Monroe Lefowitz, Robert R. Blake and Jane Srygley Mouton. "Status factors in pedestrian violation of traffic signals." *Journal of Abnormal and Social Psychology* 51 (1955): 704–706.
6. "Why people jaywalk." *Science Digest* 41 (March, 1957): 20.
7. "Curbing the jaywalker." *New York Times Magazine*, November 10, 1957, pp. 86–87.
8. Joseph C. Ingraham. "Jaywalk drive set; citizen unit to help." *New York Times*, October 4, 1957, pp. 1, 10.
9. "Just like Hicksville." *Newsweek* 52 (August 18, 1958): 32.
10. Bernard Stengren. "241 a day caught by jaywalk law." *New York Times*, August 16, 1958, p. 19.
11. Russell Davison. "On foot in the motor age." *American Mercury* 88 (January, 1959): 80.
12. Hal Tennant. "Pedestrians, arise! It's us or them." *Maclean's* 75 (November 3, 1962): 26, 48.
13. Jane Jacobs. *The Death and Life of Great American Cities*. New York: Random House, 1961, pp. 344–346.
14. Lewis Mumford. *The City in History: Its Origins, Its Transformations, and Its Prospects*. New York: Harcourt, Brace & World, 1961, p. 506.
15. "Aerial walkways: big plans for the future." *Business Week*, December 26, 1970, pp. 48–49.
16. Robert Collier and Jonas Lehrman. "The resurgence of the pedestrian." *Habitat* 16 (nos. 5–6, 1973): 28, 30.
17. Arnold W. Reitze Jr., and Glenn C. Reitze. "A place to walk." *Environment* 16 (May, 1974): 5, 43–44.
18. William Dean and Simon Breines. "Footpower in the cities." *Nation* 221 (September 27, 1975): 272, 274.
19. J. Curtis Russell, David O. Wilson and John F. Jenkins. "Informational properties of jaywalking models as determinants of imitated jaywalking: an extension to model sex, race and number." *Sociometry* 39 (September, 1976): 270–273.
20. Leonard A. Jason and Richard Liotta. "Pedestrian jaywalking under facilitating and nonfacilitating conditions." *Journal of Applied Behavioral Analysis* 15 (Fall, 1982): 469–470.
21. Kerry Diotte. "Street smarts." *Alberta Reports* 12 (February 4, 1985): 9.
22. Louis Malenfant, Ron Van Houten, R. Vance Hall and Greg Cahoon. "The use of public posting, prompting, and police enforcement procedures to increase driver yielding and pedestrian signaling at marked crosswalks." *Journal of Police Science and Administration* 13 (December, 1985): 295–300.
23. Brian Mullen, Carolyn Copper and James E. Driskell. "Jaywalking as a function of model behavior." *Personality and Social*

*Psychology Bulletin* 16 (June, 1990): 330–340.
24. "Where will we walk in the future?" *Futurist* 24 (November-December, 1990): 42.
25. Mark Bricklin. "Let's make America more walkable!" *Prevention* 43 (June, 1991): 29–30.
26. Mark Bricklin. "America wants to be more walkable!" *Prevention* 44 (March, 1992): 27–28.
27. Mark Bricklin. "America can be more walkable!" *Prevention* 44 (September, 1992): 35–37.
28. Clyde Haberman. "Going by foot, and searching for respect." *New York Times*, January 5, 1996, P. B1.
29. "Jay pride." *Economist* 346 (January 17, 1998): 27.
30. "Road and Rudy rage." *Harper's Magazine* 297 (August, 1998): 28.
31. Bill Bryson. "Out of step." *Reader's Digest* 158 (February, 2001): 71–72.
32. Nicolas Gueguen and Nathalie Pichot. "The influence of status on pedestrians' failure to observe a road-safety rule." *Journal of Social Psychology* 141 (June, 2001): 413–415.
33. Katherine Marsh. "Where 'don't walk' means jaywalk." *New York Times*, April 14, 2002, Sec 14, p. 3.
34. Ibid.
35. Marc Santora, "Etiquette of New York pedestrians is showing a strain." *New York Times*, July 16, 2002, p. B1.
36. "Living in the burbs makes us fat, study says." *Vancouver Sun*, August 29, 2003, p. A11.
37. Ibid.

# Bibliography

"Advises walking on tiptoe like gorillas to keep health." *New York Times*, August 4, 1925, p. 1.
"Aerial walkways: big plans for the future." *Business Week*, December 26, 1970, pp. 48–49.
"After hours." *Harper's Magazine* 214 (April, 1957): 84–85.
"After supper." *Times* (London), September 26, 1955, p. 9.
Allen, Robert Thomas. "Next ... automated people." *Science Digest* 53 (May, 1963): 39–41.
"An object for a walk." *Spectator* 98 (February 2, 1907): 170–171.
"And now ... the walking craze." *Marketing & Media Decisions* 21 (March, 1986): 10.
"Arrested for walking." *Literary Digest* 45 (August 3, 1912): 198–200.
Arrowpoint, Millicent. "A walking cure." *Los Angeles Times*, September 1, 1895, p. 26.
"The art of walking." *New York Times*, August 1, 1926, sec 2, p. 4.
Atkinson, J. Brooks. "Sunday morning walks." *North American Review* 217 (February, 1923): 239–246.
Austen, Ian. "Tracking your fitness, every step of the way." *New York Times*, September 20, 2001, p. C1.
Ayling, Vera. "Walking for pleasure and health." *Atlantic Advocate* 57 (August, 1967): 83.
Baker, Susan P. "The man in the street: a tale of two cities." *American Journal of Public Health* 65 (May, 1975): 524–525.
Balcom, Lois. "The best hope for our big cities." *Reporter* 17 (October 3, 1957): 19–23.
"Bayonets for pedestrians." *New Statesman* 36 (January 17, 1931): 432–433.
Beach, Stewart. "Pedestrian drift." *Atlantic Monthly* 211 (May, 1963): 114–116.
"Beauty and health report." *Glamour* 77 (April, 1979): 298.
"Bell beats Roosevelt." *New York Times*, February 6, 1908, p. 1.
Bell, J. Haslett. "The pedestrian and the city plan." *Annals of the American Academy of Political and Social Science* 133 (September, 1927): 207–214.
Berger, Meyer. "Footnotes on the pedestrian." *New York Times Magazine*, January 26, 1947, pp. 18, 48.
Blanchard, Arthur H. "Have pedestrians legal rights?" *Civil Engineering* 3 (May, 1933): 269–271.
_____. "The rights of pedestrians." *American City* 47 (November, 1932): 85.
Bleyle, Patricia Edwards. "Heavenly gait." *Ms* 17 (July, 1988): 24–25.
Blotnick, Srully. "First you put your right foot..." *Forbes* 139 (April 6, 1987): 190.
Borland, Hal. "To own the streets and fields." *New York Times Magazine*, October 6, 1946, pp. 24–25.
Breines, Simon, and William J. Dean. *The Pedestrian Revolution: Streets Without Cars*. New York: Vintage, 1974.
Bricklin, Mark. "America can be more walkable!" *Prevention* 44 (September, 1992): 35–37.

_____. "America wants to be more walkable!" *Prevention* 44 (March, 1992): 27–28.
_____. "Change your life with a walk." *Prevention* 47 (May, 1995): 15–16+.
_____. "Fix your head with walking." *Prevention* 48 (May, 1996): 25–26.
_____. "Let's make America more walkable!" *Prevention* 43 (June, 1991): 29–30.
Brien, Alan. "Afterthought." *Spectator* 212 (June 26, 1964): 866–867.
"Brisk walking eases heart disease risk for most women." *New York Times*, August 26, 1999, p. A12.
Brock, H. L. "The gentle art of walking." *New York Times Magazine*, July 12, 1942, pp. 14–15.
Brody, Jane E. "Personal health." *New York Times*, May 28, 1980, p. C10.
Bryson, Bill. "Out of step." *Reader's Digest* 158 (February, 2000): 69–72.
Carmody, Deidre. "More and more workers hit stride." *New York Times*, April 29, 1982, pp. B1, B9.
"Cheap walking." *Los Angeles Times*, April 8, 1894, p. 2.
Chrebet, Jennifer. "More ways to keep bones strong." *American Health* 14 (June, 1995): 92.
Christensen, D. "Brisk steps can reduce diabetes risk." *Science News* 156 (October 23, 1999): 260.
"City hikers." *American Magazine* 152 (November, 1951): 62.
"Citywide I.W.W. campaign." *New York Times*, December 6, 1916, p. 11.
"Closures irrelevant to railway crisis." *Times* (London), October 14, 1972, p. 5.
"Coast walk by 25,000 for Shelter." *Times* (London), April 22, 1970, p. 4.
Collier, Robert, and Jonas Lehrman. "The resurgence of the pedestrian." *Habitat* 16 (nos. 5–6, 1973): 26–30.
Collins, Glenn. "In fitness stakes, walking forges ahead." *New York Times*, May 25, 1987, p. 14.
Copeland, George H. "A curb for the jaywalker." *New York Times*, November 22, 1936, sec 8, pp. 12, 17.
Corfield, Penelope J. "Walking the city streets; the urban odyssey in eighteenth-century England." *Journal of Urban History* 16 (February, 1990): 132–174.
Cory, Christopher. "Daydreams in Manhattan." *Psychology Today* 15 (August, 1981): 16.
Cristol, Hope. "Walking: a new step for security." *Futurist* 37 (January/February, 2003): 6.
Croft, Nancy L. "Marketing." *Nation's Business* 73 (November, 1985): 33.
Cromie, William J. "Walking for health." *Saturday Evening Post* 263 (March, 1991): 68–71+.
"Crossings for pedestrians." *Times* (London), December 10, 1947, p. 2.
"Curbing the jaywalker." *New York Times Magazine*, November 10, 1957, pp. 86–87.
Dagnoli, Judann. "Walking shoes may open gait to big profits." *Advertising Age* 57 (July 7, 1986): 12+.
Davies, Hunter. *William Wordsworth: A Biography.* New York: Atheneum, 1980.
Davison, Russell. "On foot in the motor age." *American Mercury* 88 (January, 1959): 79–80.
Dean, William J., and Simon Breines. "Footpower in the cities." *Nation* 221 (September 27, 1975): 271–274.
"Decides walking is no reducer." *New York Times*, January 5, 1935, p. 19.
"The decline of walking." *Los Angeles Times*, September 18, 1896, p.10.
Deming, Seymour. "Common footing." *Atlantic Monthly* 118 (July, 1916): 72–78.
Devoe, Alan. "How to take a walk." *Reader's Digest* 34 (January, 1939): 74–76.
Dickson, Lilly. "Walking, Canada's most popular exercise." *Foresight* 8 (May/June, 1989): 34–36.
Diotte, Kerry. "Street smarts." *Alberta Reports* 12 (February 4, 1985): 9.
"Do motor cars make us lazy?" *Literary Digest* 78 (August 11, 1923): 25.
"Dr. Finley to begin drive for walking." *New York Times*, June 15, 1921, p. 4.
Donaldson, Gerald. *The Walking Book.* New York: Holt, Rinehart and Winston, 1979.
Donnan, Kristin. "Walk your way to fitness." *McCall's* 113 (June, 1986): 49.
"Drive started on pedestrians." *Los Angeles Times*, January 5, 1943, p. 2.
Durning, Alan Thein. "Pedestrian paradise." *Sierra* 82 (May/June, 1997): 36–39+.
Early, Tracy. "Test your walking I.Q." *Current Health 2* 24 (November, 1997): 20–21.

"Easing pedestrian traffic." *New York Times*, September 5, 1930, p. 22.
Easterbrook, Gregg. "Street sign." *The New Republic* 224 (March 26, 2001): 42.
"Educating pedestrians." *New York Times*, February 14, 1933, p. 14.
Eller, Daryn. "The world's easiest workout." *McCall's* 122 (March, 1995): 60.
Ellis, H. F. "Walk alone!" *Atlantic Monthly* 198 (August, 1956): 88–89.
Ellis, Rosemary. "Fitness." *Working Woman* 11 (July, 1986): 98+.
"Employees warned against jay-walking." *Safety Engineering* 70 (December, 1935): 232.
"Favor arrest of jay-walkers." *New York Times*, May 25, 1940, p. 18.
Fenn, Andrew. "The king of outdoor exercises." *American Magazine* 81 (June, 1916): 101.
"Fining the victims." *New York Times*, September 5, 1929, p. 28.
Fisher, Helen. "The way you walk that walk..." *Health* (New York, N. Y.) 21 (September, 1989): 53–55+.
Fitzgibbon, William. "Striding, the most natural exercise of all." *Reader's Digest* 100 (January, 1972): 152–155.
Flagler, J. M. "The walkers." *New Yorker* 34 (August 2, 1958): 33–34+.
"Footpath and highway." *Forum* 71 (May, 1924): 672–675.
Franks, Alan. "Oracle of the great outdoors." *Times* (London), October 15, 1983, p. 8.
Fuller, Carlos Greenleaf. "I walked a thousand miles." *American Mercury* 89 (September, 1959): 65–67.
"Futile jaywalking." *Engineering News-Record* 97 (October 21, 1926): 649.
Gale, Bill. "Talking about walking." *50 Plus* 24 (October, 1984): 62, 64.
Galub, Jack. "Walking: the most obvious and natural sport." *Glamour* 76 (June, 1978): 121, 124.
Garreau, Joel. "Don't walk." *The New Republic* 211 (September 19, 1994): 24, 28.
"Gasless." *Saturday Night* 31 (September 28, 1918): 5.
Gaynor, William J. "The pleasures and profits of walking." *Independent* 70 (June 1, 1911): 1198–1202.
Geist, William E. "A new approach to fitness chic: learning to walk." *New York Times*, February 25, 1987, p. B1.
"Gentle walking." *Times* (London), March 24, 1962, p. 9.
Gibson, Joe. "On walking." *Harrowsmith* 16 (September/October, 1991): 16–17.
"Gizmos and gadgets for walkers." *Prevention* 44 (June, 1992): 97–98+.
"Go as you please." *Los Angeles Times*, December 25, 1888, p. 5.
"Going for a walk." *New Statesman* 21 (April 28, 1923): 73–75.
Gorman, Christine. "Walk, don't run." *Time* 159 (January 21, 2002): 82+.
"Graceful walking." *Los Angeles Times*, August 11, 1883, p. 3.
Graham-Rowe, Duncan. "Tripped up." *New Scientist* 164 (December 4, 1999): 18.
"Greeks knew value of the long walk." *Science News Letter* 70 (July 21, 1956): 37.
Grice, Samantha. "The pedometer test." *National Post*, December 11, 2002, pp. B1–B2.
Groves, David. "Well-known walkers." *Good Housekeeping* 205 (October, 1987): 118.
Gueguen, Nicolas, and Nathalie Pichot. "The influence of status on pedestrians' failure to observe a road-safety rule." *Journal of Social Psychology* 141 (June, 2001): 413–415.
Gunsch, Dawn. "For your information." *Personnel Journal* 71 (February, 1992): 16, 18.
Haberman, Clyde. "Going by foot, and searching for respect." *New York Times*, January 5, 1996, p. B1.
"Half entrants finish 50-mile walk." *Times* (London), September 25, 1961, p. 6.
Hall, Carol. "Stalking walking." *Marketing & Media Decisions* 21 (November, 1986): 74–75+.
Hall, Holly. "Tired? Take a walk." *Psychology Today* 21 (May, 1987): 18.
Hambidge, Gove. "Pity the poor pedestrian." *Transit Journal* 79 (June, 1935): 172–175.
Haultain, Arnold. "Of walks and walking tours." *Atlantic Monthly* 92 (October, 1903): 476–495.
Hawthorne, Hildegarde. "A passionate walker's pilgrimage." *Century* 112 (June, 1926): 118–125.
"Heroes." *New Yorker* 58 (October 25, 1982): 40–42.

Higdon, Hal. "To your health." *Nation's Business* 76 (October, 1988): 81.
Hill, Gladwin. "Youths too soft, physicians told." *New York Times*, April 1, 1955, p. 29.
Hill, Roy. "Walking the road to better team work." *International Management* 36 (January, 1981): 32–34.
"Hit the road, Jack." *Time* 81 (February 22, 1963): 22–23.
Hocking, James H. "Do you know how to walk." *Recreation* 36 (May, 1942): 106, 114.
Hoffman, Abby. "Walk your way to good health." *Chatelaine* 52 (August, 1979): 22, 58+.
Hoffman, Harold G. "Trouble afoot." *American Magazine* 121 (February, 1936): 40–41+.
Holmes, C. N. "What walking comes to." *Scientific American* 121 (October 4, 1919): 335.
Holmes, Richard. *Coleridge, Early Visions*. London: Hodder & Stoughton, 1989.
"Hoofing it in America." *American Demographics* 18 (September, 1996): 28–29, 31.
Horsley, Carter B. "Ways of city walker detailed in study." *New York Times*, January 11, 1975, sec 8, p. 5.
"Housewives walk 3,000 miles a year in own homes, survey finds." *New York Times*, September 8, 1936, p. 29.
"How to cross a road." *Times* (London), December 13, 1938, p. 21.
"How to walk." *Good Housekeeping* 111 (July, 1940): 128–129.
"How to walk." *Good Housekeeping* 122 (May, 1946): 156.
"How to walk happy." *Better Homes and Gardens* 55 (September, 1977): 234.
"How to walk off weight." *Mademoiselle* 92 (November, 1986): 220–223.
"How, when and why you walk." *Glamour* 90 (August, 1992): 232–235.
"How women walk." *Literary Digest* 99 (November 17, 1928): 25.
Ingraham, Joseph C. "Jaywalk drive set; citizen unit to help." *New York Times*, October 4, 1957, pp. 1, 10.
Irwin, Theodore. "Let's get our feet on the ground." *Today's Health*, October, 1961, pp. 30–31+.
Jacobs, Jane. *The Death and Life of Great American Cities*. New York: Random House, 1961.
Jason, Leonard A., and Jason Liotta. "Pedestrian jaywalking under facilitating and nonfacilitating conditions." *Journal of Applied Behavioral Analysis* 15 (Fall, 1982): 469–473.
"Jay pride." *Economist* 346 (January 17, 1998): 27.
"Jaywalker guilty." *New York Times*, May 21, 1930, p. 29.
"The jaywalker menace." *Saturday Evening Post* 202 (June 28, 1930): 28.
"Jaywalking ban in effect at 8 A.M. today." *New York Times*, May 19, 1930, p. 1.
Jessup, Elon. *A Manual of Walking*. New York: E. P. Dutton, 1936.
"JFK's pace corps." *Newsweek* 61 (February 25, 1963): 23–24.
Johnson, Edgar. *Charles Dickens: His Tragedy and Triumph*. Boston: Little, Brown, 2 vols., 1952.
Johnston, Laurie. "Walk, stroll, stride, amble, but do it softly and beware of tipping." *New York Times*, April 5, 1980, p. 21.
Jonas, Steven, and Peter Radetsky. "Get in shape, go for a walk." *Redbook* 171 (June, 1988): 88–89+.
"Just like Hicksville." *Newsweek* 52 (August 18, 1958): 32.
Kahn, Carol. "Walk! It's one exercise you can do anywhere, anytime." *Vogue* 169 (February, 1979): 185.
Kay, Jane Holtz. "Without a car in the world." *Technology Review* 100 (July, 1997): 53–58.
"Keep to the left." *Times* (London), April 29, 1922, p. 21.
"Keep to the left." *Times* (London), June 7, 1922, p. 5.
"Keep to the left." *Times* (London), June 13, 1922, p. 16.
Kelly, Mae. "Walking revelations." *Hygeia* 14 (July, 1936): 625–628+.
Kerr, James. "Walking — and some of its famous votaries." *Cornhill Magazine* 154 (August, 1936): 240–245.
Kieran, John. "Out of the city, into the open." *New York Times Magazine*, December 6, 1931, pp. 12–13, 21.
King, Deborah. "Putting a swing in your step." *Times* (London), September 20, 1999, p. 55.

Kirkland, Winifred. "The wayfaring woman." *Atlantic Monthly* 109 (January, 1912): 131–135.
Kliment, Stephen A. "A view from the sidewalk." *Architectural Record* 180 (August, 1992): 9.
Kmietowicz, Zosia. "UK government urged to establish a national walking strategy." *British Medical Journal* 323 (July 7, 2001): 7.
Knight, Kathryn. "Cheat walks out of record books." *Times* (London), November 4, 1996, p. 3.
Knight, Kevin T. "Walk your way to a better body." *Better Homes and Gardens* 74 (May, 1996): 92+.
Krucoff, Carol. "Can't get to the gym? Activate your life!" *Saturday Evening Post* 270 (January/February, 1998): 26, 28.
Krucoff, Carol. "Taking exercise in stride." *Saturday Evening Post* 264 (May/June, 1992): 14, 92.
Krutch, Joseph Wood. *Henry David Thoreau*. New York: William Sloan Associates, 1948.
\_\_\_\_\_. "If you don't mind my saying so." *American Scholar* 33 (Autumn, 1964): 496–498.
Kuntzleman, Charles T. "Perfect exercise: walking." *Vogue* 172 (April, 1982): 287–288+.
\_\_\_\_\_. "Walk!—whenever ...wherever you can." *Vogue* 170 (November, 1980): 172+.
Lamb, Edward. "Weston the walker made pedestrianism a way of life." *Smithsonian* 10 (July, 1979): 89–90, 92.
Langway, Lynn. "America's foot fetish." *Newsweek* 99 (June 7, 1982): 79.
Lawless, John. "Country walks blow the cobwebs from managers' minds." *Sunday Times* (London), April 23, 1995, sec 2, p. 10.
"A league of walkers." *Playground* 19 (September, 1925): 315–316.
Lee, Rebecca E. "A prospective analysis of the relationship between walking and mood in sedentary ethnic minority women." *Women & Health* 42 (no. 4, 2001): 1–15.
Lefferts, E. B. "Effective regulation of pedestrians." *American City* 37 (October, 1927): 434–436.
Lefkowitz, Monroe, Robert R. Blake and Jane Srygley Mouton. "Status factors in pedestrian violation of traffic signals." *Journal of Abnormal and Social Psychology* 51 (1955): 704–706.
"Legs." *New Statesman and Nation* 13 (May 1, 1937): 709–710.
Legwold, Gary. "Take a walk." *Better Homes and Gardens* 77 (July, 1999): 116 I.
Le Sueur, Meridel. "The sleepwalkers." *New Republic* 75 (August 2, 1933): 313–314.
"Let's take (of all things!) a walk." *Changing Times* 26 (September, 1972): 28.
Levick, M. B. "The confusion of our sidewalkers." *New York Times Magazine*, August 3, 1924, p. 6.
Levin, Susanna. "Walking." *Health* 19 (April, 1987): 30–32+.
Lindsey, Robert. "Once upon a time, everybody walked to work; many still do." *New York Times*, November 13, 1972, p. 39.
"Line sidewalks to effect pedestrian control." *Engineering News-Record* 102 (January 3, 1929): 21.
Lippert, Joan L. "Walking!" *Family Health* 13 (June, 1981): 19–21+.
"Long walk by Y.M.C.A. man." *New York Times*, August 10, 1908, p. 3.
"Lord Grey advises British to keep their walking legs." *New York Times*, August 7, 1926, p. 1.
MacBeth, Madge. "Women I have walked with." *Saturday Night* 27 (February 28, 1914): 25.
Magennis, Mary Elizabeth. "A walker's manifesto." *Commonweal* 14 (July 8, 1931): 260–261.
Maguire, Jean. "Stroll into shape." *Redbook* 161 (July, 1983): 78–81.
Malenfant, Louis, Ron Van Houten, R. Vance Hall and Greg Cahoon. "The use of public posting, prompting and police enforcement procedures to increase driver yielding and pedestrian signalling at marked crosswalks." *Journal of Police Science and Administration* 13 (December, 1985): 295–302.
Maleskey, Gale. "Walk your way to good health." *Prevention* 38 (September, 1986): 38–40+.
"Marching back to 1066." *Life* 40 (March 26, 1956): 161–163.

Marsh, Katherine. "Where 'don't walk' means jaywalk." *New York Times*, April 14, 2002, sec 14, p. 3.
Martin, Pete. "How to walk your way to health and like it." *Saturday Evening Post* 214 (May 30, 1942): 19+.
"Mayor signs new traffic code, but rejects ban on jaywalking." *New York Times*, December 23, 1936, pp. 1–2.
McCormick, J. B. "Old-time pedestrians." *Los Angeles Times*, February 10, 1896, p. 3.
McLaughlin, Joseph. "Walk your way to fitness!" *Mother Earth News* 77 (September/October, 1982): 78–79.
Megyesy, Tim. "Reaching the fitness-walking buff through lifestyle marketing plan." *Marketing* 22 (February 15, 1988): 12.
"Men jay-walkers thrice as numerous as women." *Science News Letter* 33 (April 16, 1938): 252.
Minerd, Jeff. "Protecting pedestrians." *Futurist* 33 (August/September, 1999): 13.
"Monaghan urges daily walk to keep well during Summer." *New York Times*, June 28, 1925, sec 2, p. 1.
Montepare, Joann M., Sabra B. Goldstein and Annmarie Clausen. "The identification of emotions from gait information." *Journal of Nonverbal Behavior* 11 (Spring, 1987): 33–42.
"Motor-cars and the speed limit." *Times* (London), October 24 1929, p. 9.
Mullen, Brian, Carolyn Copper and James E. Driskell. "Jaywalking as a function of model behaviour." *Personality and Social Psychology Bulletin* 16 (June, 1990): 320–330.
Mumford, Lewis. *The City in History: Its Origins, Its Transformations, and Its Prospects*. New York: Harcourt, Brace & World, 1961.
Murphy, Suzanne. "Walk your way to physical fitness." *House & Garden* 152 (August, 1981): 28+.
Myer, Valerie Grosvenor. *Obstinate Heart: Jane Austen, a Biography*. London: Michael O'Mara Books, 1997.
Nasar, Jack L., and Kym M. Jones. "Landscapes of fear and stress." *Environment and Behavior* 29 (May, 1997): 291–323.
Nash, Eric P. "Don't walk." *New York Times Magazine*, August 29, 1993, p. 66.
Nathan, Adam. "These shoes were made for talking." *Sunday Times* (London), January 9, 2000, sec 1, p. 5.
"A new-made class distinction." *New York Times*, July 11, 1925, p. 10.
"The new walking." *Times* (London), April 1, 1938, p. 19.
Nichols, Lewis. "The light for pedestrians." *New York Times Magazine*, April 13, 1930, p. 16.
"No place for children." *Economist* 244 (August 26, 1972): 22.
"Now a clinic to teach pedestrians how to live." *Science News Letter* 34 (August 27, 1938): 141–142.
Nowell, Elizabeth. *Thomas Wolfe: A Biography*. Garden City, New York: Doubleday, 1960.
Nuttall, Nick. "Minister backs protesters who bounce cars." *Times* (London), June 6, 1995, p. 6.
"Oakland protects the pedestrian in its new traffic control." *Electrical West* 58 (May, 1927): 271.
O'Connell, George. "How to win in a walk." *New York Times*, February 3, 1980, sec 22, p. 16.
"Of walking." *Atlantic Monthly* 106 (December 1910): 856–857.
O'Hagan, Howard. "Why have we lost the joy of walking?" *Maclean's* 70 (May 11, 1957): 32, 58+.
Onativa, Elizabeth. "Pedestrian's lot not a happy one." *New York Times*, July 7, 1929, sec 9, p. 11.
O'Neill, Jeanne Lamb. "Let's take an old-fashioned walk." *American Home* 65 (December, 1962): 14–15.
O'Neill, John. "Some streets are made for walking." *New York Times*, July 23, 2002, p. F5.

"Our eight-mile daily hike." *Literary Digest* 94 (August 27, 1927): 24.
"Our point of view." *Scientific American* 160 (March, 1939): 132.
Pearson, Edmund Lester. "Walking." *Outlook* 140 (May 27, 1925): 148–149.
Peattie, Donald Culross. "The joy of walking." *New York Times* Magazine, April 5, 1942, pp. 10–11.
_____. "Walk into the world." *Recreation* 44 (May, 1950): 72–74.
Pechter, Kerry. "The first walking boom." *Across The Board* 24 (July/August, 1987): 44.
_____. "These shoes are made for walking." *Across The Board* 24 (July/August, 1987): 38–47.
"The pedestrian." *New Yorker* 39 (June 22, 1963): 19–21.
"Pedestrian League." *New Yorker* 38 (April 7, 1962): 36–37.
"Pedestrian traffic — regulation and enforcement." *American City* 36 (June, 1927): 798–799.
"Pedestrians and compulsion." *Times* (London), October 2, 1934, p. 11.
"The Pedestrians' Association." *Times* (London), November 5, 1929, p. 9.
"Pedestrians' associations." *American City* 47 (July, 1932): 68.
"A pedestrians' defence league." *Times* (London), June 20, 1925, p. 10.
"A pedestrians' defence league." *Times* (London), June 23, 1925, p. 12.
"Pedestrians get right of every which way." *Business Week*, January 5, 1942, p. 20.
"Pedestrians, our self-endangered species." *Changing Times* 33 (March, 1979): 18–19.
"The pedestrian's progress." *Times* (London), September 27, 1930, p. 11.
Pereira, Joseph. "Love blooms in the aisles." *Saturday Evening Post* 261 (September, 1989): 54–55+.
Perlmutter, Deborah E., and James H. Perryman. "How to turn your plain old ordinary walk into something sexy, assertive or athletic." *Glamour* 79 (August, 1981): 102, 109.
Pickett, Juliet B. "The witchery of walking." *Recreation* 32 (April, 1938): 9–10+.
Pierce, Bert. "Fining or jailing of jaywalkers urged by Broadway Association." *New York Times*, May 19, 1950, pp. 29, 50.
Pinkham, Mary Ellen. "The best exercise of all." *Ms* 11 (May, 1983): 59–61+.
"Poorly planned highways." *Saturday Evening Post* 206 (March 3, 1934): 22.
"Pretty soon everyone was in the act." *Life* 54 (February 22, 1963): 72A–78+.
Pringle, Murray T. "Tried walking lately." *American Mercury* 84 (May, 1957): 35–38.
"Put your walkin' shoes on, Lucy." *Broadcasting* 64 (March 4, 1963): 74.
Rader, Lloyd F. "The law of the road — traffic rights of way." *Civil Engineering* 4 (October, 1934): 515–518.
"Ramblers fight to keep paths open." *Times* (London), November 8, 1980, p. 3.
"Regulating pedestrians." *New York Times*, December 11, 1926, p. 16.
Reinhold, Robert. "Making healthful strides at area shopping malls." *New York Times*, August 13, 1986, pp, C1, C8.
Reitze, Arnold W., and Glenn C. Reitze. "A place to walk." *Environment* 16 (May, 1974): 43–44.
Rensburger, Boyce. "Pace of city life found 2.8 feet per second faster." *New York Times*, February 29, 1976, p. 46.
"Report reveals worst American cities for pedestrian safety." *Jet* 91 (April 28, 1997): 24–25.
"Reporter on a long walk." *New York Times*, May 23, 1909, sec 4, p. 1.
"A respite for jaywalkers." *New York Times*, June 2, 1930, p. 20.
"The right to walk." *New Yorker* 36 (August 27, 1960): 22–24.
"Road and Rudy rage." *Harper's Magazine* 297 (August, 1998): 26, 28–29.
"Road-hog and jay-walker." *Times* (London), November 6, 1929, p. 15.
"Road signs talk in Paris." *Times* (London), April 2, 1963, p. 11.
Rodale, Robert. "Strolling down regeneration lane." *Prevention* 40 (January, 1988): 17–18+.
Ross, Daniel Charles. "Doin' the pedestrian two-step." *Motor Trend* 39 (September, 1987): 116.
Roth, R. B. "Walk to save your life." *Safety & Health* 143 (June, 1991): 87.
Rudofsky, Bernard. *Streets for People: a Primer for Americans*. Garden City, New York: Doubleday, 1969.

"The rule of the footpath." *Times* (London), June 9, 1922, p. 15.
Russell, J. Curtis, David O. Wilson and John F. Jenkins. "Informational properties of jaywalking models as determinants of imitated jaywalking: an extension to model, sex, race and number." *Sociometry* 39 (September, 1976): 270–273.
"Safety on the roads." *Times* (London), January 22, 1938, p. 7.
Sandmaier, Marian. "Hitting your stride at noon." *Working Woman* 16 (October, 1991): 104.
Santora, Marc. "Etiquette by New York pedestrians is showing a strain." *New York Times*, July 16, 2002, p. B1.
Schmidt, K. "Stroll for health, boogie for fitness." *Science News* 140 (December 21–28, 1991): 405.
"Scientist says long walk is best election antidote." *New York Times*, November 6, 1940, p. 14.
Scobey, David. "Anatomy of the promenade: the politics of bourgeois sociability in nineteenth-century New York. *Social History* 17 (May, 1992): 203–227.
Sencourt, Robert Esmonde. *The Life of George Meredith*. New York: Charles Scribner's Sons, 1929.
Sexton, Kristy. "The death of civility." *Sunday Mail* (Brisbane), February 16, 2003, p. 30.
Shabecoff, Philip. "Germans walk, and they like it." *New York Times*, August 15, 1965, p. 72.
"Shanks' mare." *New Yorker* 39 (March 2, 1963): 23–24.
"Shank's pony." *Times* (London), September 15 1923, p. 9.
"Shank's pony." *Times* (London), April 16, 1958, p. 11.
Shapiro, Gabriel. "Watch out for drunk pedestrians." *Safety & Health* 148 (December, 1993): 100–103.
Shaw, Charles B. "Afoot in the thirties." *South Atlantic Quarterly* 20 (April, 1921): 152–164.
Shealey, Tom. "Walk your way to superhealth and slimmer hips." *Prevention* 39 (April, 1987): 66–68+.
Sheehan, Jan. "Walking: a step in the right direction." *Saturday Evening Post* 257 (November, 1985): 36+.
"Shopper's walk put at 8½ miles a day." *New York Times*, October 27, 1954, p. 32.
Siegal, Paul Z., Robert M. Brackbill and Gregory W. Heath. "The epidemiology of walking for exercise: implications for promoting activity among sedentary groups." *American Journal of Public Health* 85 (May, 1995): 706–710.
Simpson, R. E. "Pedestrian accidents." *Safety Engineering* 64 (December, 1932): 260.
"16 jaywalkers get tickets in first day." *New York Times*, May 20, 1930, pp. 1, 12.
"Some startling figures." *New York Times*, September 9, 1936, p. 26.
Spalding, Lewis A. "Take a fast walk!" *Stores* 68 (July, 1986): 25–29.
"Speaking of pictures..." *Life* 31 (October 29, 1951): 16–17.
Spearing, James O. "At the wheel." *New York Times*, January 5, 1936, sec 10, p. 6.
_____. "At the wheel." *New York Times*, May 24, 1936, sec 10, p. 6.
Spears, Tom. "Living in the burbs makes us fat, study says." *Vancouver Sun*, August 29, 2003, p. A11.
Stearns, Myron M. "Your right to cross the street." *Outlook and Independent* 155 (May 14, 1930): 50–53, 80.
Stedman, Nancy. "Learning to put the best shoe forward." *New York Times*, October 27, 1998, p. F8.
Steinhart, Peter. "The joy of walking." *Audubon* 89 (September, 1987): 8+.
Stengren, Bernard. "241 a day caught by jaywalk law." *New York Times*, August 16, 1958, p. 19.
Stephenson, Sallie. "Fitness walking for health." *Supervision* 50 (March, 1988): 9–11.
"Stepping into the beyond." *Chatelaine* 10 (February, 1937): 51.
Stockton, William. "Circling the malls to get in shape." *New York Times*, February 8, 1988, p. C11.
"Stop fake pedestrians." *Los Angeles Times*, February 1, 1914, p. ST4.
"Study shows a stroll by elderly adds years." *New York Times*, January 8, 1998, p. A15.
"Take a walk! It's good for you." *HR Focus* 70 (March, 1993): 1 sup InFocus.

"Taking a long walk." *Newsweek* 55 (January 4, 1960): 24.
"Taking a walk." *Fortune* 114 (December 8, 1986): 10.
"The talk of the town." *New Yorker* 23 (May 31, 1947): 17–18.
"Telegrams in brief." *Times* (London), February 17, 1932, p. 11.
"The telltale walk." *Human Behavior* 7 (May, 1978): 41.
Tennant, Hal. "Pedestrians, arise! It's us or them." *Maclean's* 75 (November 3, 1962): 26, 48+.
Thayer, Robert E. "Energy walks." *Psychology Today* 22 (October, 1998): 12–13.
Theodoracopulos, Taki. "Take a walk." *National Review* 45 (September 6, 1993): 71–72.
"These shoes are made for walking." *Consumer Reports* 55 (February, 1990): 88–93.
Thompson, Evan. "Walk the walk." *Canadian Banker* 101 (January/February, 1994): 10.
Thoreau, Henry David. "The joy of walking." *Saturday Evening Post* 273 (January/February, 2001). 64–66+.
"3 months to walk your way." *Glamour* 78 (May, 1980): 102.
"Through traffic." *Life* 37 (November 1, 1954): 30.
"To recapture the right-of-way for pedestrians." *American City* 68 (January, 1953): 127.
"Too many left-side walkers." *New York Times*, March 9, 1928, p. 24.
"Topics of the Times." *New York Times*, July 25, 1942, p. 12
Toufexis, Anastasia. "Make way for the mall walkers." *Time* 127 (May 26, 1986): 65.
"Tramp ends at palace." *Times* (London), March 31, 1970, p. 2.
"Transition." *Newsweek* 1 (June 10, 1933): 17.
Tucker, Larry A., and Glenn M. Friedman. "Walking and serum cholesterol in adults." *American Journal of Public Health* 80 (September, 1990): 1111–1113.
"20,000 follow in his footsteps." *American Magazine* 135 (April, 1943): 127.
"2 Marines, police clash." *New York Times*, May 7, 1944, p. 7.
Vandershaf, Sarah. "A happy pace." *Psychology Today* 21 (January, 1987): 68.
"The vanishing pedestrian." *New York Times*, January 1, 1928, sec 3, p. 4.
"The vanishing pedestrian." *New York Times*, January 4, 1928, p. 24.
Van Time, Julia. "Go the extra mile for a big healthy payoff." *Prevention* 51 (December, 1999): 48.
Vines, Gail. "The feelgood factor." *New Scientist* 158 (May 9, 1998): 53.
"Walk, do not run." *New York Times*, December 2, 1986, p. 34.
"Walk it!" *Good Housekeeping* 214 (August, 1992): 79+.
"Walk it off." *Mademoiselle* 85 (January, 1979): 58.
"Walk it off, run it off." *Mademoiselle* 88 (September, 1982): 232
"Walk Mile for Health Day is saluted by the President." *New York Times*, July 1, 1973, p. 28.
"Walk the walk." *Times* (London), July 19, 2002, p. 21
"Walk to work!" *Glamour* 80 (May, 1982): 100
"Walk to work week ends in 8-mile hike." *New York Times*, December 11, 1916, p. 6.
"Walk, walk, walk." *Newsweek* 61 (February 4, 1963): 74.
Walker, Carol Kyros. *Walking North With Keats*. New Haven: Yale University Press, 1992.
Walker, Robert Sparks. "Miles in the rain." *Commonweal* 20 (June 8, 1934): 152–153.
"The walkers." *New York Times*, April 29, 1928, sec 3, p. 4.
"Walkers are human beings." *New York Times*, December 13, 1926, p. 20.
"Walkers must be made." *New York Times*, November 16, 1909, p. 2.
"Walking, a good exercise." *Changing Times* 34 (October, 1980): 50.
"Walking: an exercise for all ages." *Consumers' Research Magazine* 65 (August, 1982): 28–29.
"Walking and character." *Los Angeles Times*, March 21, 1915, sec 5, p. 13.
"Walking as a lost art." *Saturday Night* 25 (June 22, 1912): 6.
"Walking as a punishment." *Times* (London), May 12, 1933, p. 15.
"Walking as a punishment." *Times* (London), May 22, 1933, p. 10.
"Walking backwards for a headache." *Los Angeles Times*, September 23, 1895, p. 6.
"Walking clubs are the rage." *Los Angeles Times*, February 5, 1908, p. 16.
"Walking dean." *Time* 29 (May 3, 1937): 47–48.
"Walking into shape." *Forbes* 142 (July 25, 1988): 196.

"Walking is a dangerous occupation." *Los Angeles Times*, December 16, 1923, sec 4, p. 12.
"Walking is urged as aid to defense." *New York Times*, June 18, 1940, p. 14
"Walking might help." *New York Times*, June 19, 1940, p. 22.
"Walking: Rx for better health." *Ebony* 50 (July, 1995): 56+.
"Walking shoes." *Consumer Reports* 58 (July, 1993): 420–425.
"Walking: the exercise of the '90s." *Ebony* 45 (July, 1990): 60+.
"Walking to work commendable." *New York Times*, December 7, 1916, p. 12.
"Walking up your HDL." *Prevention* 39 (May, 1987): 6.
"Walking your way to fitness." *Current Health 2* 8 (October, 1981): 15–17.
Wallace, Anne D. *Walking, Literature and English Culture*. Oxford: Clarendon Press, 1993.
Walljasper, Jay. "Mean streets." *Utne Reader*, January/February, 1994, pp. 36, 38.
_____. "Walk your talk." *Utne Reader*, November/December, 2003, pp. 6, 8.
Walmsley, D. Jim, and Gareth J. Lewis. "The pace of pedestrian flows in cities." *Environment and Behavior* 21 (March, 1989): 123–150.
"War on the roads." *British Medical Journal* 324 (May 11, 2002): 1107.
Ware, Foster. "'What good are rights?' cries the pedestrian." *New York Times Magazine*, March 18, 1928, pp. 2, 19.
"Watch your step!" *Economist* 348 (August 15, 1998): 22–23.
Watson, John S. "Cross-national studies of walking in public places." *Journal of Social Psychology* 134 (February, 1994): 119–120.
Webster, Ben. "There's a new word on the street." *Times* (London), August 28, 2001, p. 5.
Weinstein, George. "Walking for health." *Hygeia* 22 (May, 1944): 344–345+.
West, Edward Sackville. *Thomas De Quincey: His Life and Work*. New Haven: Yale University Press, 1936.
"Weston and walking." *Nation* 89 (July 22, 1909): 71.
Weston, Edward Payson. "Shanks his mare." *Saturday Evening Post* 119 (July 31, 1926): 23+.
_____. "Weston beats hoboes." *New York Times*, May 23, 1909, sec 4, p. 1.
"What your walk says about the way you think, work, love." *Mademoiselle* 85 (July, 1979): 140–143.
"Where will we walk in the future?" *Futurist* (November-December, 1990): 42.
"White lines for pavements." *Times* (London), July 3, 1928, p. 12.
White, Paul Dudley. "Walking and cycling..." *Hygeia* 15 (April, 1937): 321–322.
White, William Holly. "The gifted pedestrian." *Ekistics* 51 (May/June, 1984): 224–230.
"Why people jaywalk." *Science Digest* 41 (March, 1957): 20.
"Why walking does not reduce fatness." *Current Opinion* 73 (August, 1922): 234–235.
Wiley, John P. Jr. "Phenomena, comment and notes." *Smithsonian* 20 (July, 1989): 22–24.
Wilson, Skye. "A new road to health: walk, don't run." *Business Week*, September 26, 1988, p. 140.
Wittels, David G. "They ask to be killed." *Saturday Evening Post* 221 (January 1, 1949): 11–13+.
"Workplace walking benefits to women." *USA Today* 121 (December, 1992): 7.
Yeager, Robert C. "Walk at your own risk." *Reader's Digest* 148 (March, 1996): 187–188+.
Yordan, E. L. "For pedestrian control." *New York Times*, July 12, 1936, sec 10, p. 11.
"Young fella, walk — or wither." *America* 93 (April 16, 1955): 58.
"Youth plods along on hiking sentence." *New York Times*, January 27, 1935, p. 27.
"Youth walks 475,000 miles." *New York Times*, May 8, 1911, p. 1.
Zarrow, Susan. "Heal your heart with an easy walk." *Prevention* 40 (April, 1988): 20–24.

# Index

advertising 111–112
advice, media 53–64
aerobics 91
Afghanistan 73
Aikey, William 102
Albania 137
alcohol 140, 142,145, 164
Allen, Robert Thomas 28, 75
alone vs. companions 14, 16, 20, 41–42
American Sports Data 102
American Volksport Association 67, 116
ancient times 4
antagonism to 33
architects 81
Arnold, Matthew 20
Arrowpoint, Millicent 11
astrology 123
Athens 4
Atkinson, J. Brooks 22
Audubon, John James 16
Austen, Jane 17
Australia 51–52

Bach, Johann Sebastian 14
Bacon, Francis 13
Baker, Susan 141–142
Balboa, David 115
Balcom, Lois 141
bans, traffic 4–5
Bares, Charlie 168
Barnett, Steven 118
Bassett, David 121
Battle of Hastings 5
Baylis, Trevor 121
Beach, Stewart 49–50
Beerbohm, Max 22–23
Beihilf, Joseph 155
Bell, J. Franklin 21
Bell, J. Haslett 154

Belloc, Hilaire 20
Berger, Meyer 164–165
Berlin 32–33
Bernal, Deborah 84
Bethlehem Steel 83
bicycling 87–88
Billante, Nicole 51
blacks 84
Blair, Steven 93
Blanchard, Arthur 157
Bleyle, Patricia 83–84
Bliss, Henry 136–137
Blomberg, Richard 145
blood circulation 88
blood pressure 93, 96
Blotnick, Srully 102
bone density 95
Booton, Deborah 94
Borland, Hal 43
Bornstein, Marc H. 132
Bradbury, Ray 74
Brazil 142
breathing 61
Breines, Simon 4–5, 137
Bricklin, Mark 29, 81–82, 104, 176–177
Briffault, Robert 3
*British Medical Journal* 149
Brock, H. L. 43
Brody, Jane 29, 58, 106
Brooks company 118
Brown, Kevin 116
Bryson, Bill 29, 76–77, 177–178
business, usage of 82–83
businesswomen 46–47

Caesar, Julius 4–5
Caldwell, Bernard 164
Calgary 174
calorie burn rate 104–106
calories 62

Campbell, Ffyona 38
Campbell, Robert 9
Canada 3, 71–72, 103
cancer 95
cardiovascular system 90, 92–95
Carlyle, Thomas 15
Carmody, Deidre 75–76
Carr, Robert 112
Carter, Jimmy 44
census data 131–133
Chadwick, Henry 32
Channing, Ellery 20
children 147–148
cholesterol 93–95
cities 4, 134; dangers 148; vs. country 39–42, 79
civilization 79
class differences 5–9, 44, 72–73, 75, 133–134
clerks 130
clothing 11
clubs 31, 44, 66–71, 119
Cohan, George M. 22
Coleridge, Samuel Taylor 16–17
Collins, Glenn 115
Columbus, Ohio 164
competitions 9–10, 32
Cone, Carol 37
conflict, traffic 137, 149
Congreve, William 14
Connecticut 137
Conrad, C. Carson 100
*Consumer Reports* 106
contemplation 39–42
Contra Costa Community College (Ca.) 109
cool-downs 58
Cooper, Kenneth 91, 104
Copeland, George 162–163
Copeland, Royal S. 98

Corfield, Penelope 8–9
corporations 102
Corrigan, John 64
Coulter, John 9
Crapsey, Algernon 72
Crist, John W. 45–46
Cromie, William 31
crossings, designated 139
Crossley, J. R. 167
crosswalks 142–143, 175; UK 157–158
curative value 11
*Current Health 2* 106

Daane, Beverly 111
Dagnoli, Judann 111
dangers from walking 9
dangers to walking 138, 154, 166, 172, 176
Davies, Hunter 16
da Vinci, Leonardo 13
Davison, Russell 171
Dean, William 4–5, 137
Dear, Noach 177
death rates 92, 95
Deming, Seymour 72, 79
Denver 168–169
depression (mental) 79–80, 90
De Quincey, Thomas 14–15
Detroit 49
Devoe, Alan 53
diabetes 85
Dickens, Charles 17–18
Dickson, Lily 84, 103
Diotte, Kerry 174
distances covered 3, 5, 9, 14–23, 130, 135
dog walkers 45
Donaldson, Gerald 57
Donnan, Kristin 91–92
Doty, Alvah H. 86
Douglas, William O. 23
drive-in culture 28, 75
drop-out rates 103
Dukakis, Michael 24
Durning, Alan 147

Early, Tracy 85
Easterbrook, Gregg 148–149
eccentricity 76–77
*The Economist* 141
Eden, Emily 84
elevators 26
Eller, Daryn 106
Ellis, H.F. 41
Ellis, Rosemary 46–47, 60, 83

Emerson, Ralph Emerson 19
emotional states 1245
employees 83
endorsements 120
energy levels 125, 126
Engwicht, David 145
environmental impact 84
Erasmus 13
ethnicity 128–129
etiquette 50–52
Europeans 89
events 119
Eves, Frank 85
Ewing, Reid 179–180
excursive walking 8
exercise vs. activity 98–99
exercisers, statistics 133–135
experiments 122–128
eyesight 84

facing traffic 138
fad aspects 55, 100, 115–116
fast vs. slow walking 19, 20
Feher, Milton 58
Fenn, Andrew 78–79
50 mile hikes 35–36
Finley, John Huston 34, 67, 71
Fisher, Helen 126–127
fitness boom 100
fitness levels 88–89
Fitzgerald, George 54
Fitzgibbon, William 89–90
Flagler, J. M. 74
*Forbes* 61–62, 76
Fort Worth, Texas 156
*Fortune* 112
Foster, Edward 73–74
Frazer, J. W. 160
Fuller, Carlos 80
fur trapper 9

gadgets 64, 110, 114, 120–121
gait: recognition 122–123, 128; significance of 122–123, 124
Gale, Bill 59–60, 101–102
Galub, Jack 55, 90
Garbo, Greta 102
gasoline shortage 28
Gaynor, William J. 21–22, 25
Geisheimer, Jon 128
Geist, William 114–115
Geller, E. Scott 146
General Nutrition Centers 120

Germany 36
Gibson, Joe 81
Giuliani, Rudy 177
Gladstone, William 17
*Glamour* 56, 58, 124
Gleeson, John C. 146
Goldman, Patricia 47
golfers 130
Gondola, Joan 83
*Good Housekeeping* 46, 103
Gore-Tex 37
Gorman, Christine 65, 96
Gould, H.M. 49
Gould, Larry 83
government promotion of walking 71–72
Grey, Viscount 22
Grice, Samantha 134–135
Griffiths, David 174
Gropius, Walter 169
Gualtiere, William 55
Gulledge, Helen 107
gyms 76–77

Hall, Carol 112–113
Hambidge, Gove 159
Haultain, Arnold 39–40, 78
Havercamp, Mrs. Thomas 87
Hawkins, Francis 57
Hawthorne, Hildegarde 18
Hayes, Helen 23–24
Hazlitt, William 16
heart rate target zone 57, 59, 90
Hill, Gladwin 27
Hillaby, John 37
Hippocrates 4, 13
Hobbes, Thomas 13
Hocking, James 53
Hoffman, Abby 56–57, 99, 105–106
Hoffman, Harold 161
Holmes, C.N. 130
hostility to walking 137, 138–139, 143–144, 157, 159–160, 166–167
housewives 130–131
*HR Focus* 62–63
Huxley, Aldous 74
Hyde, Robert 92
hype 114

image of walking 7, 25, 43, 46–47, 61, 69, 72–77, 99, 100, 125–128
inactivity 100
income levels 134
Indianapolis 156
indigestion 87

# Index

indoor walking 106–109
insomnia 93
inspiration from walking 8
instructions 11, 46, 48–65
International Federation of Pedestrians 71
intersections uncontrolled 153
Irwin, Theodore 28, 41–42, 54

Jacobs, Jane 171
James, William 125
jaywalkers 151–167, 169–179; arrests 160; laws 152–153, 155–157, 177; motorist attitudes 164; and police 153, 155, 162, 164; psychology of 165, 170; shame campaigns 162, 165, 166, 167, 168
jaywalking: campaigns against 158–159; modeling experiments 169–170, 173–176, 178–179; New York City 152, 155–157, 164–166, 170–171, 177, 178–179; prevalence of 152, 169, 173, 174, 175–176, 178
Jefferson, Thomas 14
Jessup, Elon 57–58
jogging 100–102, 113, 117
Johnson, Ben 13
Johnson, Edgar 18
Johnson, Harry L. 80, 89
Johnson, Samuel 14
Jonas, Steven 60–61

Kant, Immanuel 16–17
Katz, Bruce 116
Kay, Jane Holtz 76
Keats, John 8, 15
Kelly, Mae 42, 46
Kennedy, John F. 35–36
Kennedy, Robert 35
Kent, Fred 179
Kerr, James 79
Ketchum, Bradford 74–75, 108–109, 176
King, Deborah 64–65
King, Wendy 180
Kirkland, Winifred 45
Kissinger, Henry 23
Kleinitz, Roy 148
Kliment, Stephen 81
Kmietowicz, Zosia 149
Knight, Kevin 63
Kobayashi, Shigeru 82
Komanoff, Charles 177

Krall, Elizabeth 95
Kraus, Hans 88–89
Krucoff, Carol 64, 106
Krutch, Joseph Wood 75
Kuntzleman, Charles 91, 100–101
Kunzer, Kathy 107

Laconia, New Hampshire 178
La Guardia, Fiorello 163
Lamb, Charles 14
Langway, Lynn 101
Lauer, Harvey 116
League of Walkers 67
Lebowitz, Fran 177
Lee, Rebecca 128–129
Leibel, Douglas 174
Lelyveld, Joseph 130
Leno, Jay 115
Le Sueur, Meridel 34
letter carrier 130
Levick, M. B. 48
Levin, Susanna 29, 115
Levitsky, David 92–93
Lieber, Marshall 114
lighting, street 6
Lincoln, Abraham 17
Link Up (UK) 83
Lippert, Joan 91
London 50–51
long distances 9–10, 30–38; cheating 30, 32–33, 37–38; 50-mile hikes 35–36; marketing 37; political uses 36–37; UK 35, 36–37
longevity 89–90, 101–102
Loren, Ivan 155
Los Angeles 99, 152–153, 162, 164

machinery 26
*Mademoiselle* 55–56, 59, 60, 123
Magennis, Mary 27
Maguire, Jean 101
Maimonides 13
Malenfant, Louis 175
mall, pedestrian 178
mall walking 106–109
managers 82–83
Mansfield, Mike 72
marathons 33–34
Marckx, Mary 114
marketing 37, 110–121
Marsh, Katherine 178–179
Martin, Pete 53
math calculations 59, 60, 104–106, 133–134

McAdoo, William 138, 155
McAughey, T. J. 30
McBeth, Madge 41, 45
McKinlay, Arthur Patch 4
McMurray, Helen 52
McNutt, Paul 74
McShane, James 179
media outlets 35–36
medical care system, costs 104
meditation 80
Meeker, Ezra 26
Megyesy, Tim 120
Mercer, Frank 35
Meredith, George 18–19
Middle Ages 6–7
Minneapolis 172
mockery of walking 114–115
Moffat, John 146
Monaghan, Frank J. 87
Montepare, Joann 125
moods 85, 124–126, 128–129
Moore, Barbara 35
Moreno, Rita 115
Moritz, Carl Philip 7
motorists 145, 171
movement therapy 64, 127
Muir, John 16
Mullen, Brian 175
Mumford, Lewis 5–6, 171–172
Munsell, Suki 64
Murphy, Suzanne 99–100

National Highway Traffic Association 153–154
National Sporting Goods Association 112
National Walking Week 104, 115
negligence 157, 172–173
New Delhi, India 144
*The New Statesman* 137
New York City 6, 71
*New York Times* 71, 74, 130–131, 137
Nichols, Lewis 154
Nietzsche, Friedrich Wilhelm 20–21
night walks 15, 17, 23, 42
Nike 112, 113, 118
Nixon, Mark 128
Nixon, Richard 72
Norris, Steven 69
Nowell, Elizabeth 23

Oakland 152
obesity 86–87, 94–95, 179

## Index

obstacles to walking 141, 179–180
O'Connell, George 28–29
O'Leary, Dan 33
Onativia, Elizabeth 41
O'Neill, Jeanne 75, 80
Oparowski, Paul 119
O'Toole, Peter 24
outfits 114–115, 118
overpasses 143, 172

pace 18, 23, 61–63, 89, 95–96, 98, 117
Pakradoonian, George Jr. 114–115
Parry, H. C. 51
Paulin, Borisse 90
Pearson, Edmund 73
Pearson, Lester 26
Peattie, Donald 79
Pechter, Kerry 10, 115–117
Pedestrian League of America 69–70
Pedestrians' Association 68, 157–158
Pedestrians' Protection Association 68
pedometers 120–121
Penfield, Wilder 72
Penn, William 14
peripatetic school 4
Philippe, Louis 25
Phillips, Lewis 49
philosophy of 39–47
physicians 27
Pickett, Juliet 79
Pinkham, Mary Ellen 59
planners, city 142, 146, 148, 179–180
Plato 13
Pliny the Elder 4
Plowden, Ben 69
Pocock, Hubert 87
police reaction 74, 99
Polk, Richard 113
Pollack, Michael 100
Pompeii 5
Powers, Rich 110–111
powerwalking 23, 102
President's Council on Physical Fitness and Sports 72, 90, 101
prevalence of walking 25–29, 99–104, 113, 117, 133–134
*Prevention* 119
Pringle, Murray 27, 54, 89
Pritikin, Nathan 91
promenading 4, 8–9
Proxmire, William 23, 72

psychology of 122–129
public relations firms 115
Puma company 111
punishment, walking as 73–74
Pyke, Richard 7

Raben Publishing 110–111
Rader, Lloyd 158
Rath, Julius 30–31
recklessness 160
Reclaim the Streets 69
Reebok 116
Reeves, Steve 23
regulations, public relations 152–153, 160–162, 170–171
Reinhold, Robert 107–108
Reitze, Arnold 172
Reitze, Glenn 172
Replogle, Michael 145
retail outlets 113–115
Rippe, James 91, 94, 126
Ritter, Don 177
Robarge, Maurita 123
Robinson, John 109
Rockport 37, 111, 112, 114, 116–117
Rodale, Robert 80–81
role models 119–120
Roosevelt, Theodore 21, 67
Rosario, Raymond 115
Ross, Daniel 143–144
Rousseau, Jean-Jacques 14, 82
Rudofsky, Bernard 6, 99
Ruskin, John 21
Russell, Bertrand 57
Russell, J. Curtis 173

safety issues 134
Salinger, Pierre 36
San Francisco 163, 168
Sandmaier, Marian 62
Santora, Marc 50
school students, bussed or driven 29
*Scientific American* 139
Scobey, Davis 9
Scott, Walter 17
Seattle 162
self-esteem 83
Sellers, Peter 89
Sencourt, Robert 18–19
Shabecoff, Philip 36
Shakespeare, William 13
Shelley, Percy B. 17
shoe makers 111–121
shoes 11, 56–57, 76; athletic 111; purpose-made 57, 60, 103–104, 108, 111

shoppers 130
shopping centers 104–106
Shoup, David M. 35
sidewalks 143, 172, 178; lanes 49
Sidgwick, Arthur 41
sing test 59
skin conditioning 88
Smith, Charles E. 73–74
Snodgrass, Sara 124–125
socks 54
solitude 78
Spalding, Lewis 112
Spearing, James 138–139, 159–160
Spears, Tom 179–180
spectators 34
Sproul, Arthur 49
standards 62–64, 91–92, 96
statutory control 141
Stearns, Myron 156
Stedman, Nancy 127–128
Steinhart, Peter 44–45
Stephenson, Sallie 82–83
Stevenson, Robert Louis 20
Stockton, William 108
Stoic philosophy 4
Storie, Catharine 34–35
Storie, Thomas D. 34–35
Straus, Jack 170
street access, common law 156
streets: congestion 4–5, 49–50; instruction to cross 174; layout 5; right vs. left side 48–52
stress levels 93, 126
stride 62–63
strolling 80–81
studies, research 92–95
style of walking 45–46, 56
suburbia 75, 134, 147, 172, 179–180
supervisors 82–83
Surface Transportation Policy Project 147–148
Sweetgall, Robert 37, 102
Swift, Jonathan 14
sympathy to walkers 140

talk test 59, 63–64
10,000 step program 121, 134–135
Tennant, Hal 171
Terry, Luther L. 36
Thailand 145
Thayer, Robert 85, 125, 126
therapeutic value 81–82, 115
thinking 14, 20–21, 22, 79–80

Thompson, Evan 95
Thompson, W.H. 79–80
Thoreau, Henry David 19–20
Thurrot, John 165
Tilly, George 43
*Times* (London) 9, 28, 68
Toufexis, Anastasia 107
traffic: separation 140–141, 143, 169, 171; signal timing cycles 147, 153, 159, 168–169, 171, 174; signals 152–153, 168–169
traffic accidents: ages 141; costs of 146; day vs. night 137; death rates 136, 180; drivers not charged 146; fault of 136, 138, 139–140, 179; lack of media attention 148; Rio de Janeiro vs. Baltimore 142; statistics 137, 140, 144, 146, 147, 148, 149, 160, 177
transit strike 29
transportation: options 26–27; system design 142; to work 131–134
travel books 7
Trevelyan, George Macauley 21
Truman, Harry S 23
types of walking 42, 101, 115, 123, 124, 127

underpasses 159

United Kingdom 50–51, 68–69, 73, 83, 128, 141, 149, 157–158
urban sprawl 148, 179

Valentine, Lewis J. 160
Veblen, Thorstein 75
Vickies, Joan 69
victims, blamed 140, 142–143, 145
Vines, Gail 85

Waldorf, Lynn 99
Walker, Carol Kyros 15
Walker, Robert 42
*The Walking Magazine* 110–111
Walkways Center 119
Wallace, Anne 6–7
Walljaspar, Jay 82, 145–146
Walton, Izaak 15
Ware, Foster 154
warm-ups 55
Washington, D. C. 161–162, 166
Watson, John 52
weight reduction 87, 104–106
Weight Watchers 102
Weinshall, Iris 178
Weinstein, George 88
Wepman, Joseph 170
West, Edward Sackville 14–15

Westinghouse company 158–159
Wesley, John 14
Weston, Edward Payson 10, 31–32
whistle test 59
White, Gilbert 15
White, Paul Dudley 87–88, 90
white lines 49
Whyte, William 143
Wichita, Kansas 139, 166
Wilensky, Leo 69–70
Wiley, John P. Jr. 84
Wilkinson, Bill 147
Wilkinson, Jody 95
Williams, Jack 30
Wilson, Skye 102–103
Winnipeg 171
wisdom 79
Wittels, David 139–140
Wojecki, Eddie 99
Wolfe, Thomas 23
women 45–47, 51, 75–76, 87, 128–129
Wordsworth, Dorothy 16
Wordsworth, William 16
World War II 53

Yeager, Robert 146
Yordan, E. L. 160–161

Zale, Matt 114

www.ingramcontent.com/pod-product-compliance
Ingram Content Group UK Ltd.
Pitfield, Milton Keynes, MK11 3LW, UK
UKHW041959140426
5217IPUK00015B/877